Smart Guide™
to
Getting Strong and Fit

About Smart Guides™

Welcome to Smart Guides. Each Smart Guide is created as a written conversation with a learned friend; a skilled and knowledgeable author guides you through the basics of the subject, selecting out the most important points and skipping over anything that's not essential. Along the way, you'll also find smart inside tips and strategies that distinguish this from other books on the topic.

Within each chapter you'll find a number of recurring features to help you find your way through the information and put it to work for you. Here are the user-friendly elements you'll encounter and what they mean:

The Keys
Each chapter opens by highlighting in overview style the most important concepts in the pages that follow.

Smart Money
Here's where you will learn opinions and recommendations from experts and professionals in the field.

Street Smarts
This feature presents smart ways in which people have dealt with related issues and shares their secrets for success.

Smart Sources
Each of these sidebars points the way to more and authoritative information on the topic, from organizations, corporations, publications, web sites, and more.

Smart Definition
Terminology and key concepts essential to your mastering the subject matter are clearly explained in this feature.

F.Y.I.
Related facts, statistics, and quick points of interest are noted here.

What Matters, What Doesn't
Part of learning something new involves distinguishing the most relevant information from conventional wisdom or myth. This feature helps focus your attention on what really matters.

The Bottom Line
The conclusion to each chapter, here is where the lessons learned in each section are summarized so you can revisit the most essential information of the text.

One of the main objectives of the *Smart Guide to Getting Strong and Fit* is not only to better inform you about how to start an exercise program, but to make you smarter about how to incorporate fitness into your day in a safe, gradual way to ensure a lifetime of healthful benefits.

Smart Guide™

to

Getting Strong and Fit

Carole Bodger

CADER BOOKS

John Wiley & Sons, Inc.

New York • Chichester • Weinheim • Brisbane • Singapore • Toronto

The information contained in this book is not intended to serve as a replacement for professional medical advice. Any use of the information in this book is at the reader's discretion. The author and the publisher specifically disclaim any and all liability arising directly or indirectly from the use or application of any information contained in this book. A health-care professional should be consulted regarding your specific situation.

Library of Congress Cataloging-in-Publication Data:
Bodger, Carole.
Smart guide to getting strong and fit / Carole Bodger.
p.   cm.   — (Smart guide)
Includes index.
ISBN 0-471-29635-X
1. Physical fitness—Popular works. 2. Exercise—Popular works. 3. Weight lifting—Popular works. 4. Reducing exercise—Popular works. 5. Aerobic exercises—Popular works. 6. Health—Popular works. I. Title. II. Series.
RA781.B59   1998
613.7—dc21   98-33833

Printed in the United States of America

10 9 8 7 6 5 4 3 2 1

Contents

Introduction

Fitness is not something reserved for the bodybuilder, the Olympic athlete, the supermodel, or the young. Fitness is a healthy state of mind and body that everyone can—and should—claim.

In this book we hope to help you do just that. In chapters 1 and 2 we introduce the overall concept of fitness, the many ways in which it can be measured, and how to recognize those that apply to you. By helping you to set realistic fitness goals tailored to your own needs, desires, and capabilities, and sharing some strategies on how to stay motivated along the way, we hope to provide you with a good start on the journey to a fitter, healthier life.

Chapter 3 looks at the three dimensions of a complete fitness program—aerobic or cardiovascular exercise; anaerobic or strength training; and flexibility work—with specifics on how to apply each for a balanced workout plan. In chapters 4 and 5 we weigh the pros and cons of working out at a gym and on your own, with recommendations on how to get the most from either tack.

The next few chapters provide the latest word on good nutrition for every healthy body, with special attention to the exerciser's needs; and an exploration of the ever-growing number of alternative approaches to better health, from movement therapies and meditation to acupuncture and massage. We conclude by taking it all on the road—into the workplace and our favorite restaurants, to airports and hotels, on vacation, onto the playground and ball field—into real life, where fitness belongs, every day.

If there's anything we want this book to convey it's that fitness isn't a thing separate and apart from "real" life. To the contrary, by being integrated into our daily way of living, the fitness lifestyle makes life far better than it otherwise could be.

Before undertaking any program that calls for a significant change in your activity level or dietary intake, of course, check with your physician. Then go out and live!

CHAPTER 1

....

The First Step

To be "fit," the dictionary tells us, is "to be appropriate, prepared, competent, adequate; adapted to an intended end or purpose; suitable by nature, character or circumstance." Each of us has our own personal definition of fitness; an individually tailored and refined standard that suits our bodies and our lives. Establishing that personal standard goes a long way toward helping us measure, and attain, our own "perfect fit."

Fitness Defined

Our standard of physical fitness is based on health, not athletic ability. We define fitness as the ability to perform daily activities with vigor. Health-based fitness comprises three broad components. All are important and weakness in any one throws the wellness equation off balance.

1. Cardiovascular fitness. This essential component of health is the ability of the heart and circulatory system to get oxygenated blood to the muscles so that the body can produce energy. It is also known as cardiovascular endurance, cardiorespiratory fitness or endurance, or aerobic fitness. The better you can do that, the longer and better your life will be. Good cardiovascular fitness reduces the risks of atherosclerosis and heart disease, diabetes, certain types of cancer, and numerous other health-related ills.

2. Musculoskeletal function. This combines muscle strength and endurance with flexibility, and can be well appreciated by the 80 million Americans whose day-to-day movements are hampered by chronic low-back dysfunction. Fitness in this area has been estimated to prevent up to 80 percent of backaches. Maintaining good musculoskeletal function can also slow muscle deterioration and the lessening of bone density that occurs with age, reducing the risks and severity of osteoporosis and extending and improving quality of life into our older years.

3. Body composition. Of greater importance than how much we weigh is body composition, or the proportion of lean muscle tissue to fat tissue, often referred to as the percentage of body fat. By maintaining weight that's lean in nature (that is, weight that is not excessive in body fat but that is composed of lean muscle tissue, which supports proper body functioning and contributes to optimal health) we can reduce our risk of the many health hazards associated with obesity, including prolonged stress on the heart, hypertension, and respiratory problems. Being too lean, however, can also be a problem; at extreme levels it causes bone loss and an increased likelihood of fracture.

Each of the three aspects of physical fitness has its own particular requirements, though improvements in one area will ultimately benefit the other two. The better your musculoskeletal function, for instance, the more easily and effectively you can perform the sort of exercises that strengthen your heart and reduce the percentage of body fat.

Proper nutrition, adequate rest, and a contented state of psychological well-being are keys to health, wellness, and overall physical fitness. However, as our lifestyles have become increasingly sedentary, more and more studies now recognize the importance of physical activity. Indeed, remain-

SMART SOURCES

Those with concerns related specifically to the elderly will find these organizations valuable resources:

American Association of
  Retired Persons
601 E St., N.W.
Washington, DC 20049
800-424-3410
www.aarp.org

National Council on the
  Aging
409 Third St., S.W.
Washington, DC 20024
800-424-9046
www.ncoa.org

National Institute on
  Aging Information
  Center
P.O. Box 8057
Gaithersburg, MD 20898
800-222-2225
www.nih.gov/nia

ing active is so inexorably linked to wellness that fitness and activity have become practically interchangeable concepts.

In the summer of 1996, the landmark *Surgeon General's Report on Physical Activity and Health* concluded that regular moderate physical activity, expending as few as 1,000 calories per week, can reduce the risk of developing or dying from some of the leading causes of illness and death in the United States, including heart disease, diabetes, high blood pressure, and colon cancer. "The good news is you don't have to train like an Olympic athlete to enjoy the benefits of a healthy lifestyle," said Donna E. Shalala, Secretary of the U.S. Department of Health and Human Services, who commissioned the study. Acting Surgeon General Audrey F. Manley called the report "nothing less than a national call to action."

Moderate regular physical activity was found to reduce feelings of depression and anxiety; to help control weight; to aid in building and maintaining healthy bones, muscles, and joints; to enable older adults to become stronger and better able to move about without falling; and to promote psychological well-being. It also has been linked to reduced risks of breast cancer as well as osteoporosis. In addition, it increases dexterity, endurance, and strength; improves the quality of our sleep; enhances the ability to perform daily tasks; boosts immune systems; and strengthens resistance to injury. Its benefits cut across many different areas of life, by improving mood, sharpening intellectual skills, lowering health-care costs, and contributing to a better social life.

And it can do so well into old age.

How to Tell If You're Fit

Sometimes it may seem that depending upon whom you talk to—and what chart you look at—you can find yourself more or less physically fit. Talk to one person and "you're fine" if your weight is in a certain proportion to your height and build. Talk to another and you have nothing to worry about as long as your heart rate and blood pressure are at certain levels. Talk to others and it's your fat-to-muscle ratio, or your percentage of body fat; still others measure fitness in terms of agility, strength, or endurance. One thing for certain in the view of most health professionals is that there's controversy here.

If you remember that physical fitness involves three basic components and not just one, you can keep those one-dimensional standards in their proper place. There are many standards and modes of measurement, and many are applicable. To be truly fit requires a combination, a balance. If your weight is "correct" but your body is a collection of flabby tissue, you have room for improvement. If you're toned but your heart races after a leisurely stroll, or if a visit to the doctor's office reveals that your blood pressure is soaring above 120/80, you have a way to go.

"Your aerobic fitness level, not your body weight, is the best measure of your overall health," according to Steven N. Blair, P.E.D., senior scientific editor of the 1996 Surgeon General's report. "In terms of health and longevity, your fitness level is far more important than your weight."

F.Y.I.

• 58 million adults—over a third of the adult U.S. population—are overweight or obese.*

• 25 percent of American adults do no exercise at all.**

• Regular moderate physical activity (using 150 calories a day, or 1,000 calories per week) can substantially reduce the risk of heart disease, diabetes, colorectal cancer, breast cancer, high blood pressure, depression, and anxiety.**

* Shape Up America!

** *Surgeon General's Report on Physical Activity and Health*

Cardiovascular Fitness Measurement

Cardiovascular, or aerobic, fitness is measurable via stress tests performed by or in the presence of a physician as you walk a treadmill. Stress tests monitor your heart rate and blood pressure as you go from a resting state to maximal levels of exertion.

A submaximal, or submax, test might be performed at a gym or health club, and it evaluates your heart at the lower levels that are considered your aerobic exercise target zone—about 50 to 85 percent of the maximum heart rate, or pulse per minute, for your age (the maximum is roughly

How Much? How Often?

All or nothing has sent many well-intentioned fitness-seekers to the sofa. From making the gym a home-away-from-home, to hitting your cardiac target three times a week for thirty minutes, to just moving a little bit more as often as you can handle it, we've all heard a different version of "proper dose."

The latest school of scientific thought offers good news: Regular moderate physical activity offers substantial benefits in health and well-being for the vast majority of Americans who are not physically active. And that can mean expending as few as 1,000 calories per week. For people who are already moderately active, greater health benefits can be achieved by increasing duration, frequency, or intensity at a gradual pace.

For optimal health benefits, the generally accepted recommendation is to try to get a minimum of thirty minutes of moderate-intensity exercise almost every day of the week at 60 percent of your maximum heart rate (subtract your age from 220 and multiply the result by 0.6). And that thirty minutes need not be taken all at once: Studies confirm that three sessions of ten minutes can be just as effective, resulting in a significant impact on weight and health.

The indisputable fact: Anything is better than nothing.

calculated by subtracting your age from 220). Blood pressure levels, which are best measured by a doctor's rather than on frequently faulty self-test machines, are indicated with two numbers, the top number (systolic blood pressure) measuring pressure as your heart pumps blood and the bottom (diastolic blood pressure) measuring pressure when your heart is relaxed. The lower your blood pressure, the easier it is for the heart to function. Levels are considered high at 145/95, the generally accepted indicator of hypertension.

Musculoskeletal Strength Measurement

Musculoskeletal function is also measurable by fairly universally accepted tests. However, like all the tests described here, these are used to attain baseline or starting points from which to measure your progress, not to attain absolute figures. Flexibility tests examine the degree to which you can stretch various muscles groups. Strength tests can be static, in which you push or pull against an immovable fixture; or dynamic, in which you manipulate a movable weight in various ways. Endurance tests look at the length of time at which you can perform a variety of physical exercises.

Body-Composition Measurement

Measuring body composition (or body fat) is at the forefront of most dieters' lists of concerns.

The methods of measurement vary greatly, in regard to accuracy, cost, and test complexity.

The most accurate (if cumbersome) strategy involves taking your weight while you are submerged underwater. Because muscle is more dense than fat, the more muscle you have, the deeper you'll sink and the more water you'll displace. The new-to-the-market Bodpod chamber works on the same theory, measuring air instead of water displacement.

While both of these methods tend to be expensive and are available only in sophisticated health-care and personal-training facilities, many health clubs and weight-loss programs measure body fat via the use of skinfold calipers, which pinch and measure the thickness of fat at various body sites. Bioelectric impedance analysis involves sending a small electric current through the body; the more fat, the slower the current will flow. But while both approaches can be effective, they can both yield inaccurate results if the subject is severely obese or underweight, or if they're performed by an inexperienced tester—like the newest hire at the gym, which wants you to buy its fat-reducing services.

Other, more accessible, methods are the most popular. Weight-for-height charts of generally acceptable weight guidelines might take frame, age, and gender into account; or they might not. And they don't differentiate fat from muscle (which weighs more).

Body mass index, or BMI, used for decades by the medical and obesity research communities, can be a valuable measure of weight-related disease risk—it's the measure used in most studies. A ratio between height and weight, BMI also provides a generally reliable measure of body fat for the average sedentary American on the average American diet. It is not, however, reliable for competitive athletes or bodybuilders, whose BMI is high due to a relatively larger amount of muscle; women who are pregnant or lactating; growing children; or the frail elderly.

To calculate your BMI, multiply your weight (in pounds) by 703. Next, multiply your height (in inches) by your height (in inches). Lastly, divide the answer in step 1 by the answer in step 2. For example, a woman who weighs 120 pounds and is 5 feet tall is at mimimal health risk.

$$120 \text{ pounds} \times 703 = 84{,}360$$
$$5 \text{ feet} \times 12 \text{ inches a foot} = 60 \text{ inches}$$
$$60 \text{ inches} \times 60 \text{ inches} = 3{,}600$$
$$84{,}360 \div 3600 = 23.43$$

High BMI levels can indicate an increased risk of developing diseases such as hypertension, cardiovascular disease, adult-onset diabetes, sleep apnea, osteoarthritis, and female infertility; a BMI over 30 usually is considered a sign of moderate to severe obesity, with all its inherent concerns.

The BMI measurement poses some of the same problems as the weight-for-height tables. Not all doctors agree on the cutoff points for "healthy" versus "unhealthy" ranges, and BMI does not provide specific information on percentage of body fat.

Body Fat Distribution

Not only does the quantity of fat matter, but so does its location. Men usually carry theirs around their stomachs or abdomens, giving them what's known as an apple shape. Women tend to amass

F.Y.I.

With the public's increased interest in fitness comes an increase in the number of people and organizations hawking wares. Beware of the following:

• Advice to buy a product from an individual who would profit from its purchase.

• Claims of 100 percent effectiveness or zero side effects.

• Claims that deficits in one area of wellness (nutrition, fitness, exercise, and so on) are responsible for all of your life's ills.

• Studies consisting of small groups of people, groups that don't include people like you, or that don't mention the number or type of people being studied.

• The use of testimonials rather than properly designed and documented scientific studies.

Are You at Risk?

BMI	Health Risk
Less than 25	Minimal
25–26	Low
27–29	Moderate
30–34	High
35–39	Very high
40 and higher	Extremely high

their extra weight in the hips and buttocks, for a pear shape. Of course there are exceptions. Some men are pears and some women are apples—especially after menopause. Apples are at greater risk of developing the health problems associated with obesity.

To measure whether you're an apple or a pear, calculate your waist-to-hip ratio: Measure the waist at its narrowest point, then measure the hips at their widest, then divide the waist measurement by the hip measurement. Women with ratios greater than 0.8 and men with ratios greater than 1.0 are apples and, what's most important, at increased health risk.

Setting Realistic Goals

Some of us can pump up to a size akin to Mr. Universe, run a four-minute mile, show off cellulite-free thighs, keep our heart rates at a steady fifty beats per minute, and live to be one hundred.

Most of us can't.

Pursuing unrealistic or inappropriate goals, such as losing more weight than is medically advisable or lifting more weight than your spine can support, will result in disappointment—which can turn the most earnest seeker of fitness away from any exercise at all. It can also result in physical harm or injury to your body.

Setting achievable goals means taking into

account what's most important to you and what's possible for you, and then developing a workable fitness routine.

"Most people are not going to expend more than 300 or 400 calories per session," notes Randy Claytor, Ph.D., senior adviser to the President's Council on Physical Fitness and Sports. "And you know how little it takes to put that many calories into your mouth."

There are some things that exercise can do for us and some that it can't. Unfortunately, the people who sell us videos, gadgets, and other infomercial schemes and paraphernalia—with their bulging muscles and buns of steel—are prime examples of the latter. "Those bodies," Claytor reminds us, "aren't going to happen to 99.9 percent of us no matter what we do."

The factors to consider when establishing your goals can be divided into two basic groups: "Your Givens," what you're born with and what you're living with now; and "Your Variables," what you're willing—or are able—to control and vary to achieve your goals.

Your Givens

Age

Although it is never too late to set out on a program of better physical fitness, in general the later in life you begin, the more distance there may be to travel. The more years of couch-sitting, car-riding, elevator-riding (in other words, sedentary) living you have behind you, the more of an adjustment you'll be asking your body to make. Changes in bone density, the flexibility of aging

SMART SOURCES

Organizations that can provide useful health and fitness information related to women are the following:

The Melpomene Institute for Women's Health
1010 University Ave.
St. Paul, MN 55104
612-642-1951
www.melpomene.org

National Women's Health Resource Center
5255 Loughboro Rd. N.W.
Washington, DC 20016
202-537-4015
www.healthywomen.org

tendons and ligaments, and a slower metabolism also need to be taken into account. So when you read in *Men's Health* that "the average guy" can run a mile in twelve minutes, remember that may mean an average between guys who are approaching their golden years and guys in their teens.

Physical Condition at the Start

If your job plants you behind a desk for eight hours a day, the chances are you'll be less physically limber than a kindergarten teacher who runs after toddlers five days a week. Similarly, those who are setting out on a fitness program because their doctor has warned them about cardiovascular disease or to strengthen their abdominal muscles after a bout with lower-back pain are not advised to set the same goals as those in better health.

Gender

As equal as we should be in the workplace, men and women are far from equal when it comes to their needs in the workout room. From recommended body fat levels (men shouldn't drop below 3 percent or exceed 20 percent body fat; women shouldn't fall below 11 percent or surpass 30 percent), to different levels of strength, we are, simply, different. Fitness goals must reflect as much.

Body Type

In the 1940s, William H. Sheldon presented his theory of "somatypes," three basic, genetically determined body types that he linked with certain personality traits. Reference to these body types today is more likely to be found in the gym than the psychologist's office, but somatypes are still credited with affecting physical potential in various ways. Ectomorphs, characterized by delicate build, low body fat level, high metabolism, and a small amount of muscle mass and muscle size, are suited to endurance athletics but might find it a challenge to gain weight and muscle mass. Mesomorphs, with a medium-to-large build, low-to-medium body fat, a medium-to-high metabolism, and a large amount of muscle mass and size, can aim for power athletics and tend to have no trouble gaining or losing weight. Endomorphs' large build bears a high percentage of body fat and underdeveloped muscles that can be developed with relative ease, although a slow metabolism makes losing weight a challenge.

Your Variables

Time

The number of hours you have available to devote to reaching your goals is important to keep in mind before you set those goals. If your high school reunion is coming up next week, it's not wise to set your heart on being ten pounds lighter in time to impress the campus queen or king. If you're a tax accountant, think twice about your goal of investing an hour at the gym every night as the calendar nears April 15. Or if you simply find your life dishes out the proverbial "full plate"—family and friends, choir practice, household chores, bowling league, and your weekly stint at the local soup kitchen—the stress imposed by a rigorous exercise regime is likely to result less in workout than in burnout.

SMART SOURCES

Getting heart-healthy and in shape is one of the hardest things you'll ever do in your life! Let these organizations help you in your efforts:

American Heart
  Assocation
7272 Greenville Ave.
Dallas, TX 75231
214-373-6300
800-242-8721
www.amhrt.org

Shape Up America!
6707 Democracy Blvd.
Suite 306
Bethesda, MD 20817
301-493-5368
www.shapeup.org

Effort

Although the popular "no pain, no gain" philosophy should be regarded as potentially harmful, the goals you are able to accomplish do bear a direct relation to the amount of effort you are willing to expend. Stretching tendons, increasing your lung capacity, running a mile all involve a lot of effort. You'll breathe harder, sweat more, and—especially at the start—sometimes wake up a little sore the morning after.

Commitment

To find the time and exertion that are involved in reaching the loftiest goals takes a strong foundation of commitment. And that's not likely to exist if your goals have more to do with satisfying someone else's expectations or desires, or filling a need that is more appropriately addressed in, say, a marriage counselor's office than in a gym. A healthier, stronger, more physically fit body will reward you with numerous social as well as physical benefits—the better you physically feel and the more comfortable you are with your physique, the more easily you'll be able to share that happiness with others—but if you're looking for love rather than longevity, social acceptance rather than strength, it's best to look elsewhere.

Finding the Right Approach

The proper fitness strategy is different for everyone, depending upon many variables: your goals, reasonably set (weight loss, increase in endurance, strength); your personality; where you're starting from; your lifestyle; your likes and dislikes; your current energy level; and so on. Do you have the time to invest to look like Xena, Warrior Princess? Do you have the dedication it takes to become a marathon runner? Do you have the physique to become an Olympic gymnast? Do you enjoy the feeling of clean, strong lungs more than cigarette smoke?

Before starting, it's important to learn what kinds of physical activities are appropriate to attain your particular goals. If you want cardiovascular benefit, for instance, sprinting isn't the answer; in this case, running more slowly would speed your way to aerobic health.

• **For those more interested in toning and shaping than in bulking mass,** the best plan would emphasize repetition rather than exertion; more whole-body aerobic exercise, such as swimming, and less weight training.

• **For the overweight,** calorie-burning activities in combination with diet are the proper tack. A continuous but not too strenuous workout that uses large-muscle groups will bring healthy, gradual results. As the weight comes off, the strategy can be adjusted to tone and shape.

• **For the young,** with growing bones and skeletal structure, care is advised—unbalanced training that overly develops one muscle group over another can lead to deformity. Sports and athletic games provide a well-rounded workout, developing cardiovascular and pulmonary strength, stimulating circulation to benefit muscle growth, and

SMART MONEY

"Keep a simple log of how much time you spend being active and being inactive," says Andrea L. Dunn, Ph.D., of the Cooper Institute for Aerobics Research. "Use a step-counter to count steps and see how many you get in in a day. If you can get about ten thousand steps in a day, you'd meet minimal public health guidelines for physical activity."

improving bone density. Youth is also the time for an early introduction to proper warm-up and stretching routines.

• **For the elderly,** care must be taken to protect brittle bones and stiff joints, and attention must be paid to the many other factors that can affect strength and balance. It's important not to stress tendons and ligaments or the cardiovascular system beyond a safe target level. Low-impact exercises such as water aerobics provide a great starting point; an underwater environment provides smooth resistance that guards against quick accelerations and decelerations, which can cause harm.

• **For bodybuilders,** very specialized weight-lifting routines are prescribed to maximize muscle mass, density, and definition, using a variety of exercises with every muscle group imaginable. A combination of heavy weights and moderate-to-high repetitions is often combined with a specialized high-protein, high-carbohydrate diet.

• **For the physically challenged and those with chronic, disabling conditions,** physical activity can improve stamina and muscle strength. Exercise can be obtained via longer sessions of moderately intense activity (thirty to forty minutes of movement in a wheelchair) or shorter sessions of more strenuous activity (twenty minutes of wheelchair basketball).

For *everyone,* doing too much too fast means running the risk of getting hurt, or physically or emotionally drained, and giving up altogether. A good idea for beginners might just be to spend some time reading up on proper fitness routines before undertaking them, while implementing moderate lifestyle changes that incorporate more physical activity into the daily routine.

James R. Morrow Jr., Ph.D., professor and chair of the Department of Kinesiology, Health Promotion, and Recreation at the University of North Texas in Denton, points to Americans' increasing body weight as a key marker of our decreasing fitness. According to Centers for Disease Control and Prevention statistics for the years 1988 to 1994, 34.8 percent of adults between the ages of twenty and seventy-four are considered overweight, 10.4 percent more than in the years 1960 to 1962.

"Any amount of physical activity expends calories and is cumulative," says Morrow. Indeed, research has shown that significant changes in lifestyle activity alone can result in improvements in cardiovascular fitness, musculoskeletal function, and body composition—and the accompanying lowered health risks that they imply—in amounts statistically equivalent to those experienced by people in a structured exercise program. And they have a slightly greater likelihood of keeping you at it for longer periods of time (see chapter 2).

Staying Motivated

The rewards of reaching a goal and seeing your fitness efforts produce results provide powerful motivation that can spur you on to even greater progress. Eventually, you establish a routine that works for you and becomes part of your life. In short, once you understand how to do it and get

SMART SOURCES

Here are helpful organizations for those with special needs:

National Organization on Disability
910 Sixteenth St., N.W.
Suite 600
Washington, DC 20006
202-293-5960
www.nod.org

National Spinal Cord Injury Association
8300 Colesville Rd.
Suite 551
Silver Springs, MD 20910
301-588-6959
800-962-9629
www.spinalcord.org

Special Olympics International
1325 G St., N.W.
Suite 500
Washington, DC 20005
www.specialolympics.org
202-628-3630
800-700-8585

U.S. Disabled Athletes Fund
2015 South Park Pl.
Suite 180
Atlanta, GA 30339
770-850-8199
www.gsu.edu/~wwwusd/usdafvi.htm

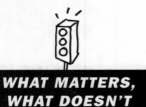

in the habit of doing it, your success encourages you to continue doing more.

Yet many of us throw in the proverbial towel before reaching that stage. "Sixty percent of the people who start out drop out before that point where they've gained some benefits and gain that intrinsic reward," says Randy Claytor. And remember, when you get that reward depends on your fitness level at the start, your age, your body type, and many other factors. To keep fit means keeping at it. No matter how good any program is, it's no good at all if you give up.

Here are some suggestions to help you stay motivated:

• **Go public.** Announce your intentions—and successes—out loud. People who care about you will be encouraging, and those who don't are likely not the sort of positive influences you want in your life. Friends, family, and coworkers will ask you about your progress as you go along; some might even offer useful hints they've found helpful in their own lives. Just be wary of those who try to force their own way of doing things on you. Everyone's an individual.

• **Proceed slowly but surely.** Don't overdo it. You can hurt yourself physically and frustrate yourself mentally. If your body isn't used to strenuous movement, or maybe any movement at all, the impact of starting out full throttle can be damaging. You hurt yourself, you get frustrated, you stop. One strategy is to start with small changes in your activity level throughout the day—take the stairs, park the car farther away, walk more. Start out easy and work up. And never get to the point where your routine takes over your life.

• **Enjoy yourself.** Doing what you like to do provides the best motivation of all. Work out your muscles in a way that isn't torture. Taking a walk can provide more interesting scenery than you'd get while tallying your miles on a treadmill. Playing a game of basketball or another sport can be a winning strategy for combining fun and health.

• **Don't go it alone.** Enlist a friend. Not only will you gain the pleasures of companionship, and the boon of sharing progress with each other along the way, but by making a commitment to another person, you can bolster your commitment to yourself.

• **Choose your surroundings.** Don't work out in a place you hate to be—whether that means the gym, your dusty basement, or a track in a dangerous part of town. What's appealing to someone who enjoys the social aspects of a gym might mortify another who prefers a more private space.

• **Forget the fast results.** At the start, after establishing your baseline measurements, don't even look at a scale or tape measure. You might be disappointed, and less likely to go on. Fitness takes time. Give yourself a lot of it.

• **Don't compare your progess with that of others.** Even on identical fitness programs, different people get different results. Some start out strong and plateau. Some maintain a gradual pace all along. Others seem to have nothing happen and then suddenly make a major leap. Those who start out with a lot more to accomplish will also be more likely to see results faster, simply because there's that much more to do. Many factors are at work: your diet, health status, medications, your state of

STREET SMARTS

Steven Pacino, a thirty-eight-year-old paralegal whose work load was sapping the energy he used to spend on exercise, discovered the benefits of having a workout buddy: "I used to break a sweat kicking the kickstand out. Since my partner and I started bicycling together, I've been able to do about five miles a few times a week after work and on weekends—and keep at it."

THE BOTTOM LINE

Being physically fit is not an absolute or all-or-nothing proposition, but a personally defined and constantly evolving state of health. The three main components—cardiovascular fitness, musculoskeletal fitness, and body composition—each contribute to our overall well-being, and combined with proper diet, rest, and emotional nourishment, account for a better quality of life. By increasing daily activity by even moderate amounts, most men and women can decrease the risk of life-threatening disease, reduce stress levels, and attain a broad range of other benefits. If we set realistic, achievable goals appropriate to our individual needs, desires, and abilities, physical fitness is within our reach.

mind. Keep a personal log to measure your own progress against your own starting point.

• **Stay entertained.** Invest in a portable radio or Walkman, a good book, even a tiny TV. Working out should be fun and relaxing; boredom and drudgery are not part of the plan. Find good music with a stimulating beat. Get a book with a good binding that lays flat on the equipment; a large-print edition is even better.

• **Schedule wisely.** The time at which you exercise, as well as the days you choose to do so, can make a difference. Don't plan to work out when you're exhausted after the office, or when the kids are clamoring for dinner, or when it's the only time that you and your nonexercising spouse have to yourselves. But do allocate time on a regular basis—consider it an appointment with yourself.

• **Reward yourself.** Set moderate, measurable, attainable short-term goals and reward yourself when you reach them—with a new outfit, tickets to a concert or a sporting event, a day at the spa.

• **Believe in yourself.** Believe you can succeed. "Research shows that believers are far more likely to be successful than doubters," says Barbara J. Moore, Ph.D., president and chief executive officer of Shape Up America!, an organization founded by former Surgeon General C. Everett Koop in response to America's "obesity epidemic." "You really have to take a look at your attitude toward your objectives and whether you believe you can reach them." If you think you can, chances are you will.

Staying on Track

A body at rest will resist being set in motion. So states the Law of Inertia. And when it comes to our bodies, that law too often applies.

No matter how well our minds understand the benefits of fitness, no matter how many studies or statistics we read, our bodies may need some prodding to get in gear. Starting out with a sensible plan that takes into account our needs, our goals, our abilities, and our objections can help clear the obstacles to which we're so ready to surrender—and help us get (and stay) on track.

Prescreening for Exercise

Any reputable fitness plan will carry a "Contact your doctor before starting an exercise program" disclaimer. The warning is sometimes less altruistic than it is mandated by corporate lawyers worried more about legal liability than your health.

True, there can be some risks involved. Extreme physical activity can cause musculoskeletal injuries, and the chances of having a heart attack if you're not careful are greater during physical activity than they are while you're lounging around watching TV. The sudden death of runner Jim Fixx was all that many reluctant exercisers needed for them to say, "I'm safer on the sofa." But you're not. The overall risk of a cardiac emergency is low—about one death per 400,000 hours of jogging, even lower in those who exercise regularly—and is far outweighed by the overall health benefits and disease-prevention boons of exercise.

Testing that involves mild exertion, common-sense caution, and self-administered questionnaires are the best way for healthy people (from adolescence to early old age) to gauge readiness for a low- to moderate-intensity exercise and fitness program.

The current standard is the PAR-Q (Physical Activity Readiness Questionnaire), developed in Canada decades ago and widely accepted in the United States. The American College of Sports Medicine recommends the seven-question survey specifically for healthy men over forty and women over fifty. Those who answer yes to any of the questions are advised to check with a doctor first.

The trouble with PAR-Q: "We were getting rather many people who were responding positively to the original questionnaire when in many cases there was no problem," says Roy J. Shephard, M.D., Ph.D., D.P.E., of the University of Toronto. "The biggest issue had been that a physician sometime in the past had said they had high blood pressure, although if they were the type of person who became nervous the first time they put their nose inside the doctor's office, that itself could be the cause."

Shephard and two of his colleagues reworded the PAR-Q to be more inclusive, and the President's Council on Physical Fitness and Sports now recommends the revised version (rPAR-Q) as the method of choice for determining exercise readiness in "symptom-free adults with no more than one major cardiac risk factor"—such as smoking, excessive intake of alcohol or caffeine, or drug use; high blood pressure or cholesterol levels; or a high body mass index (BMI).

Some people shouldn't need the test to know a doctor's consultation is in order: those who have been diagnosed with heart disease, arthritis, diabetes, or respiratory ailments; or who have allergies, leg cramping, or feel pain when exerting themselves. So should anyone who is pregnant or has a family history of sudden death at a young age. And if you have a cold, flu, or just

Revised Physical Activity Readiness Questionnaire (rPAR-Q)

1. Has a doctor said that you have a heart condition and recommended only medically supervised activity?

2. Do you have chest pain brought on by physical activity?

3. Have you developed chest pain in the past month?

4. Do you tend to lose consciousness or fall over as a result of dizziness?

5. Do you have a bone or joint that could be aggravated by the proposed physical activity?

6. Has a doctor ever recommended medication for your blood pressure or a heart condition?

7. Are you aware through your own experience, or a doctor's advice, of any other physical reason against your exercising without medical supervision?

If you answer no to all the questions, you can be pretty sure that you can start becoming much more physically active—begin slowly and build up gradually. If you answer yes to one or more questions, talk with a doctor first. It doesn't mean you shouldn't increase your physical activity or that you won't benefit from it, only that you might have to avoid certain types of exercise or should start off at a slower pace. By being aware of specific areas of risk, you can be more alert to warning signs.

don't feel well, don't exercise until you feel better.

In most cases, the health risks of inactivity far outweigh the risks of an exercise program. Shephard agrees with Swedish physiologist P. O. Åstrand: He would sooner order a medical examination for somebody who wasn't going to exercise than for somebody who was.

The Basics

Anyone who tells you that physical activity—or anything else—alone is all you need to live to be one hundred is making a bit too much of a good thing. A good exercise routine is simply a good health habit that is buoyed by other good health habits and in turn, bolsters them. Feed your body properly and you'll have more energy to work out; work out properly and you'll find you're sleeping better; get better rest and you'll be better able to cope with mental stress; live a serene lifestyle and your body can process nutrients better. Likewise, deficits in one area will hamper the others. Don't feed yourself properly and your body won't be able to produce the energy it needs to exercise; exercise too much and you'll deprive your body of important rest; overtax yourself and your immune system will be weakened, leaving you susceptible to a wide range of illnesses. Each aspect of health is related to the others.

Health-Risky Behavior

• Undertaking a much more intense activity than you're used to, or doing it for a longer period of time than you're used to.

• Working out under time pressure or emotional stress.

• Heavy lifting or prolonged extremes of muscle contraction.

• Allowing competition, publicity, or pride to keep you going despite warning signs.

• Exercising in extremes of heat or cold.

• Exercising when you don't feel well.

Nutrition

A varied, moderate, and balanced eating plan that supplies the right amount of nutrients and energy is essential for achieving and maintaining strength, flexibility, and endurance. In a later chapter we address the body's need for specific vitamins and minerals, and the best ways to get them. But how we consume them has a lot to do with health—not only because we can help our bodies process the nutrients better (we can absorb only so much vitamin C at a time, for instance), but because certain strategies can help keep us on track.

The latest research is leaning away from the "three squares" to the "grazing" approach: Smaller meals, four to six times a day, give the body a more consistent supply of fuel.

"Eating something every three hours keeps blood glucose levels in the body and brain at more consistent levels," says Leslie Bonci, R.D., of Allegheny General Hospital in Pittsburgh, and a spokesperson for the American Dietetic Association (ADA). And that keeps our bodies energized and our minds sharp. Also, by lessening the chance that we'll be "starving" before our next meal, it can help us to eat more sensibly and be less frantic about food preparation, making the meal more pleasant and easier to digest.

If you're working out, eating a reasonably sized, balanced meal of protein, carbohydrate, and fat three hours beforehand allows enough food to support your efforts, and enough time to process it so that you don't have a full belly weighing you down. For early-morning exercisers, a light carbohydrate-based snack—a piece of toast or a handful of dried cereal—an hour beforehand is a good idea.

To keep your body hydrated during activity, the ADA recommends four to six ounces of fluid (four to six gulps) every fifteen to twenty minutes. And afterward, don't fast. Experts suggest you have a light carbohydrate-and-protein snack within thirty minutes of working out to replenish your stores.

"If we are going to command something from our body demanding energy expenditure, we want to make sure that we're giving our body enough to go on," says Bonci.

Rest

"Good health requires good sleep," Quentin Regestein, M.D., states matter-of-factly in *Sleep Problems and Solutions.* But the amount of sleep we need per night varies so much from person to person, and at different stages of our lives, that putting a number on how many hours we should get could keep anyone tossing and turning all night long. Suffice it to say: If you find yourself yawning through the day, you need more.

Mental Attitude

Rest also means relaxing while awake. Our lifestyle may be sedentary, but even with all that lying around, our minds continue to race. We have bills to pay, families to attend to, bosses who are impossible, and thanks to the Internet, information overload follows us into our homes. We can all take a tip from the twelve-step groups' Serenity Prayer: Seek the serenity to accept the things you cannot

Sleep Tips

To Get to Sleep More Easily:

• Don't try to force it.

• Don't eat a heavy meal before bedtime.

• Cut back on caffeine, alcohol, and tobacco consumption.

• Don't read suspense thrillers in bed.

To Get a Better Sleep:

• Invest in a quality mattress and bedding.

• Make your bedroom a stress-free zone; keep tension-producing objects and tasks—like work—out.

• Don't sleep with the television on.

• Pull the shades.

change, the courage to change the things you can, and the wisdom to know the difference.

Bringing art and fresh-cut flowers into your life, saying grace before meals, and taking "news fasts" are some of the life-enhancement strategies advocated by popular New Age health guru Andrew Weil, M.D. Soothing music, candlelight, and long baths have long been chicken soup for mental duress. Simply put, a peaceful environment brings us peace. Physical activity also has been shown to reduce stress levels (but worrying over how much physical activity we get will not).

Medical Care

Regular annual checkups at the doctor and dentist keep us up-to-date on our physical health in ways we cannot always evaluate ourselves. And the sooner problems are detected, the less damage they can do. Get your teeth cleaned. Have your eyes checked. The American Cancer Society recommends that beginning at age forty, women have an annual mammogram; men a digital rectal exam. Beginning at age fifty, both men and women should have yearly tests for colorectal cancers, and men also should have an annual-prostate specific antigen blood test. People at different levels of risk have different needs. Consult a physician for the right schedule of preventive care.

Establishing a Baseline and Gauging Progress

To gauge your progress, you have to establish a baseline of starting measurements, which will give a good, personal comparison point. Some of those measures (blood pressure, cholesterol count) can be found in the results of your latest physical. Others you can take yourself: weight; body mass index (BMI); the measure of your chest, waist, hips, and thighs; the amount of weight you can lift without strain; the number of miles you can comfortably walk; how long you can sustain a muscle stretch.

Although your resting pulse—the rate at which your heart beats normally—isn't going to change dramatically, monitoring your heart rate during exercise can provide a good objective measure. To take your heart rate manually, touch the first two fingers of one hand to the pulse site at the base of the thumb of the other hand, or to the carotid artery at the side of the neck. Count the number of beats over a ten-second period, and multiply by six for your beats per minute (bpm). Many exercise machines have monitors built into the hand grips or on attachable chest straps, and there is a wide variety of accurate ear-clipped and fingertip pulse meters, among others. All will measure your heart rate for you, and can be easier to deal with than taking your own pulse during exercise. Ranging in price from $60 to more than $400, body-worn monitors come in over fifty different varieties.

Remember, the standard estimated target heart rate zone (50 to 85 percent of the figure you get when your age is subtracted from 220) is an estimate, with an error rate of plus or minus twelve beats. When you're gauging progress, compare yourself with yourself.

Subjective versus Objective

There are many things that are measurable, and then there are some important ones that are not.

In the beginning, objective measure—the things you can count (heartbeats), weigh (overall pounds), tally (inches), and gauge with a meter (blood pressure)—is likely your best bet, because your progress, especially at the start, will—and should—be too gradual to readily detect. It's encouraging to see you've lost a pound when a look in the mirror might not show it, and the littlest bit of progress can motivate you to keep up the good work.

But in the long run, subjective self-evaluation—how you look and feel—is the best indicator of success. Objectively measured changes may taper off (your blood pressure can only get so much better), while the subjective measures (increasingly greater energy) continue on.

Feeling more comfortable in a smaller size of clothing, for instance, can be more relevant than what you learn from the scale alone. Muscle has about three times the density of fat, so as you begin to gain muscle mass and lose fat, your progress might not be evident in the number of pounds you weigh.

Also, objective measures aren't much comfort if you aren't able to appreciate how the weight loss or improved heart function affects your day-to-day life. Looking better and feeling better count far more than any numbers alone can convey.

One good subjective measure, rate perceived exertion (RPE), involves a personal assessment of your exercise intensity—in other words, the feelings caused by your exertion during a workout or other physical activity. These sort of feelings, says the American Council on Exercise, will reflect the combined input of muscles and joints; breathing rate, heart rate, and other metabolic processes; as well as psychological and environmental factors. RPE is usually assessed on a 0 (no exertion at all) to 10 (maximal exertion) scale. Resting, for instance, would have a rating of 0; walking at a pace that feels moderate for you would be a 3; running uphill might be a 10. The recommended RPE range for most people during exercise is usually between 3 (moderate) and 5 (strong). At the beginning, you might rate walking a fifteen-minute mile as a 4; after a week of walks, you might experience the same pace as a 3 or 2. And that's progress.

Personal Logs

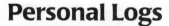

Personal logs of both objective and subjective accomplishments can be extremely helpful devices for keeping track of the strides you're making, assessing your progress toward short- and long-term goals, and seeing whether your approach is working for you. Keeping a record of what you do, and what it's doing for you, offers a psychological boost that can be motivating as well.

"It's important to keep track because it adds a little bit of ritual to it," says Richard Cotton, an exercise physiologist with the American Council on Exercise. "Personal logs help you look at success, and get it out of the head and into a physical form in the world."

F.Y.I.

Children today spend an average of seventeen hours a week watching TV, in addition to the time they spend on video and computer games. They are heavier and less physically fit than children were even a generation ago and showing early signs of cardiovascular disease.

Source: American Heart Association

There are many preprinted exercise logs on the market, with varying degrees of detail to be recorded over a variety of periods of time. Those designed for runners, for instance, focus on mileage covered, duration, and speed, while those for weight-lifters have columns for pounds lifted, number of repetitions, and length of time spent on sets. Beginners might find the sheer number of listings off-putting, and might prefer developing a log of their own. Using more visual graphs or bar charts, as opposed to referring to lists of numbers, lets you see your progress at a glance. The main thing is to make your "personal log" just that. Use the method that feels right for you, with an amount of information that doesn't overwhelm.

"Some people are simply 'list people,' and they operate differently," says Cotton. "For them, recording a lot of detail can actually become more of a hindrance than a help."

Above all, don't confuse keeping your log with actually doing the exercise. If you forget to write down an activity, that doesn't mean it doesn't count. "An evening walk that isn't recorded," Cotton reminds us, "is still an evening walk."

Determining Your Course of Action: The Best-Laid Plan

After you've looked carefully at yourself, your needs, and what you're able and willing to give in terms of time and energy, and you've set your goals sensibly, taking your baseline and medical status into account, you have all you need to develop a plan of attack. Think of having a specific strategy as a road map toward your goals. Not only will it better help you reach them, but you won't have to wake up in the morning and wonder what you'll have to do that day to get there—or allow room for the possibility that thinking about how you'll exercise is as far as you'll get. Write it all out beforehand in your log and reevaluate periodically. A good routine isn't static but changes to suit your changing needs.

Making the Time

The time you have available will determine what you can do with it. If you have one hour open after work on Mondays, Wednesdays, and Fridays, you might plan a program of stretches combined with aerobic and anaerobic activity for each session, putting your focus on different areas of the body on different days. If you're starting out with ten-minute exercise breaks in the course of your daily routine, you might stretch in the morning, take a brisk walk in the afternoon, and do some strength training at night. (Just don't plan to do any of this at a gym that takes twenty minutes to get to.) The point is to distribute a variety of workout activities into the time periods you're able to set aside. If you plan an ambitious program but don't have the time required, you're setting yourself up for failure from the start.

SMART MONEY

For a good visual record of when you work out, post a calendar in your kitchen or office and mark your exercise days with gold stars or brightly colored stick-on dots. Says Richard Cotton of the American Council on Exercise, "It's like an award."

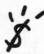

Optimal Payback

For optimal exercise benefits, consult your internal clock. Circadian rhythms, the daily cycles that our bodies follow, regulate everything from metabolism to blood pressure, and their influence on body temperature has been found to have an effect on workout quality. When body temperature is at its highest—usually late afternoon, between four and six o'clock—exercise is most productive. To determine your own circadian peak, record your temperature every few hours for five or six consecutive days (look for plus or minus 1.5-degree changes throughout the day). Try exercising anywhere from three hours before to three hours after the time at which you register your highest temperature. Depending on whether you feel most energetic in the morning or night, you might find your temperature peaking an hour or two before or after the norm. Those in training for a specific athletic event should train at the time of day for which the event is scheduled.

Whatever you do, don't change a schedule that works for you for one that's an intrusion in your life. Any time is better than nothing at all. If you feel good beginning your day with exercise (and people who exercise in the morning have been shown to be better at keeping it a habit), keep at it. Just be sure to allow yourself more time for warm-ups and stretching to ready your body for action.

Plan for the Year

Adjust your program over the course of the seasons. Don't plan an outdoor walking program in the winter if you live in the North or in the summer if you live in the Deep South—neither is good for your health and both will detract from your enjoyment of the activity. Instead, take your walk at the mall or on a treadmill. When short winter days allow less daylight time for that outdoor after-work basketball game, check out a neighborhood recreation center's facilities.

Equipment and Clothing

Especially at the start, there's no need to buy a thousand-dollar weight-lifting system or make a major investment in designer exercise togs . . . unless you're the type for whom a financial commitment provides the proof—and motivation—you need to make a serious investment in getting fit. If you're not, such unnecessary expenditures can merely be draining, and too many well-intentioned beginners have found themselves saying, "Forget the exercise—I've exerted myself enough."

Once you establish a program and know what range of activities is involved, you still need to know what particular equipment suits your personal abilities, preferences, and tastes. You can use what's available at a gym, or local fitness or recreation center; consider rentals; or even find a less equipment-based approach that can provide you with the same results as a pricey machine.

The clothing you wear should be comfortable (physically and in terms of how you'll feel to be seen in it if you're working out in public), and not restrict or inhibit movement. Look for fabrics that are easy to care for, and provide adequate ventilation to allow sweat to escape. If you'll be outdoors, it's a good idea to have at least one garment

SMART SOURCES

American Council on Exercise
5820 Oberlin Dr.
Suite 102
San Diego, CA 92121
619-535-8227
www.acefitness.org

Solid advice on a wide range of fitness topics, with a referral line to qualified professionals in your area. "Fit Facts," helpful tip sheets on everything from ab crunches to yoga, are available through an automated phone system at no charge by calling 888-FIT-FAXX (888-348-3299).

equipped with a hood. If you'll be in the cold (and that includes overly air-conditioned gyms), dress in layers to stay warm—but not too warm: Overheating puts undue stress on the heart.

A dizzying array of sports footwear offers support of all kinds, appropriate for the stress exerted on different areas of the foot during dif-

Warming Up and Cooling Down

Taking a few minutes to warm up before and cool down after exercise can radically improve results. Not only does a warm-up improve calorie-burning and ready you mentally, but it prevents cardiovascular problems; improves the elasticity of joints and muscles, thereby helping to prevent injury; and improves performance by giving you better muscle control. In short, it allows you to work out more safely, more comfortably, and more effectively.

There are two phases to both warming up and cooling down: aerobics and stretching. The first few minutes should be spent in light aerobic exercise that uses the muscles you'll be using during your workout—a sort of slow-motion version of your planned routine. If you're preparing for a walk, for instance, simply start out by walking at a slower pace. If you'll be lifting weights, arm and upper-body movements are

appropriate. Continue until you feel slightly perspired, but not tired out.

Once you've completed the aerobic warm-up—literally warming the temperature of the muscles and so increasing their elasticity and resistance to harm—take the time to gently stretch the muscles you'll be working out. Start each stretch slowly, deeply exhaling and inhaling as you gently stretch the muscle. Try to hold each stretch for at least ten to thirty seconds, and don't bounce or hold your breath. For morning workouts or those performed in colder weather, warm up longer.

It is just as important to cool down afterward. In something of a reverse of the warm-up, gradually decrease the intensity of whatever you're doing. Stopping too quickly may make you pass out or get dizzy or nauseated, and can have harmful effects on the heart. A series of stretches can prevent next-day soreness and injury.

ferent activities. Start off with a good, basic, cross-training shoe and a good pair of insulating socks. A more detailed discussion of equipment and clothing can be found in later chapters.

Working Out How You'll Work Out: The Exercises

A good overall fitness program has three major components: aerobic activity for cardiovascular endurance and fat burning, anaerobic activity to build strength (both described in detail in the next chapter), and flexibility training to increase your range of motion and lower your risk of injury.

• **To improve your cardiovascular system, increase your metabolism, burn body fat, and build endurance,** try aerobic physical activities such as brisk walking, running, bicycling, swimming, line dancing, hiking, or cross-country skiing, to an extent that brings you into your target heart zone (50 to 85 percent of your maximum heart rate). A low- or no-impact aerobic activity that you can sustain for at least thirty minutes a day is recommended for those who want to lose weight.

• **To build muscle strength, tone up, promote leaner body mass, and increase bone density,** try anaerobic routines such as weight training, sprinting, and exercises like push-ups, crunches, dips, and leg lifts. Unlike aerobic training, which can

STREET SMARTS

Two women, two ways:

Susan Thor, a thirty-five-year-old Fort Lauderdale horticulturist who spends her days planting and climbing trees, gets her physical activity on the job and her serenity from weekly massages and after-hours drives in her vintage Triumph. A self-professed "chocoholic," she hasn't had a weight problem in years.

Rosalind Hartz, a thirty-eight-year-old office worker in Tulsa, gets her exercise at the neighborhood fitness center three days a week, on the steps to her high-rise apartment, and on walks with her dog. "If I didn't plan to get some activity in, my bottom would be shaped like an office chair."

be thought of as a body-wide approach to fitness, anaerobic activity strengthens and tones specific muscles.

• **To improve flexibility and posture, reduce the risk of injury, increase physical and mental relaxation, and release muscle tension and soreness,** stretching is crucial. One of the most often overlooked and misunderstood aspects of fitness, stretching is often thought of merely as part of a warm-up or cool-down routine—a sort of bastard child of the aerobic/anaerobic team. The truth is, stretching is the foundation on which the others can be built. Ideally, every part of the body should be put through a full range of motion in the course of a day, although doing so within the span of a week is certainly acceptable. It is crucial to flex the muscles in those areas you'll be working out during any other routine. Different stretches are good for different activities. Runners should stretch their lower back, the muscles in the back of the thighs and calves, and the inner thighs. A racquetball player should stretch those same leg muscles, as well as the muscles in the upper back, shoulders, and neck.

Whatever your goals, wherever your emphasis, a good fitness plan will include a variety of exercises for different parts of the body. Don't just work out your upper or lower, front or back—an imbalance can result in more damage than no workout at all. A fitness appraisal by a certified exercise physiologist or personal trainer is an excellent way to determine your basic fitness and what will help you most.

Everyday Exercise

Thanks to the Surgeon General's report, we now have the government's word that when it comes to physical activity, little things can make a big difference. By incorporating painless changes into our daily routine, we can significantly improve our health.

There's a lot to work with. The modern conveniences that were to have blessed us with a life of ease have cursed us with the risks such a sedentary lifestyle can hold. Automatic doors open for us; remote controls let us remain inert on the couch; the Internet makes it possible to shop, go to work, educate ourselves, find entertainment, and even conduct an active social life without ever leaving the computer screen; dishwashers wash and dry; voice-activated word-processing programs even let us write without lifting a finger to a key.

Any amount of physical activity expends calories; any use of muscles will help maintain strength. Resisting the seductive lure of all those nasty energy-saving shortcuts, carrying a little bit of extra weight (balanced on both sides), or standing while you're waiting for an appointment are some of the things that can add up to a healthier life.

Project Active, a study of 235 healthy but inactive men and women, compared such a "lifestyle physical activity" approach with a structured exer-

Warm Up First

Before doing any stretching, start out with low-level aerobic exercise, which literally warms you up by increasing the temperature of your muscles and making them more pliable. (You'll notice it's much easier to stretch after a warm shower or a soak in a hot tub.) To be most effective and help prevent injury, the stretch should be held—not bounced—for a period of ten to thirty seconds or longer, as you exhale through your mouth, then inhale deeply through your nose. Don't stretch a muscle that isn't warmed up; don't strain; and don't hold your breath.

What to Expect

• **Evolution.** Your fitness routine isn't static. Think of your body as a sculpture. The first few months you're knocking away huge hunks of stone, then comes the fine-tuning and detail work. As you go along, evaluate, appraise, and refine to reflect your changing goals and abilities.

• **Impatience.** Nothing happens overnight. Waiting for results can be frustrating, but overexuberance is dangerous. Losing weight, increasing strength—it all takes time.

• **Aches and pains.** Especially for the previously inactive, microscopic tears in newly stretched muscles can cause next-day soreness and tightness. A proper warm-up and cool-down can minimize the damage and the pain. Discomfort that persists or incapacitates you is a warning sign that you're doing too much or doing it improperly.

cise program to compare the subjects' physical changes and cardiovascular disease risk factors.

Men and women between the ages of thirty-five and sixty were randomly assigned to either the structured exercise group, whose activities were gymnasium-based; or the lifestyle group, given relatively free rein to decide how they wanted to increase their activity levels. Several men who worked sitting at computer terminals for most of the day, for example, programmed their machines to beep reminders of break times for activity; some took longer routes to the office copy machine. One woman enlisted social support by starting a walking club at her church.

At the end of six months, both groups had achieved a greater level of cardiorespiratory fitness and increased their use of behavior strategies, and both had statistically equivalent decreases in blood pressure and percentage of body fat, according to Andrea L. Dunn, Ph.D., associate director of the Division of Epidemiology and Clinical Applications at the Cooper Institute for Aerobics Research in Dallas, who worked on the study.

As for who tended to stick with the program: After an eighteen-month follow-up, Dunn said that "we have some evidence that the lifestyle group did a little better, although [the results are] not as clear-cut as we expected."

The conclusion: Both structured and lifestyle approaches can work.

Use the following as some ideas to get you jump-started to incorporating more activity in your daily life:

Around the House

• Do strenuous housework—vacuum the floors, clean the windows, dust and wash the walls and ceilings.

• Hide the remotes—get up to turn the stereo or TV on or off, or to change the channel.

• Forget the riding mower; use the push-and-pull type.

• Bathe and groom Fido, then take him for a long walk or run.

• Use that cordless and walk around when you're on the phone.

In the Kitchen

• Empty the contents of your cabinets, wash everything, then rearrange it all, putting some things out of reach so you'll have to stretch or climb occasionally.

• Pass up the salad-in-a-bag; buy fresh vegetables and wash and prepare them yourself.

• Scrub and polish your appliances.

WHAT MATTERS, WHAT DOESN'T

What Matters

• Finding out if you're at risk of harming yourself before starting and exercise program.

• Choosing a well-balanced approach to health.

• Warming up and cooling down.

• Staying in touch with your progress.

What Doesn't

• What time of day you exercise or where you do it.

• The bathroom scale.

• Expensive equipment and designer workout clothes.

• Excruciatingly detailed fitness logs.

At the Office

• Take the long way to the copy machine.

• Don't use the automatic doors; use your arm muscles.

• Never sit for more than thirty minutes at a time.

• Do some stretches or adbominal exercises in the privacy of your office.

On Your Way

• If you can't walk all the way there, walk to the train or bus.

• Get out a stop earlier.

• Park the car at the far end of the parking lot.

• Take the stairs.

• When you walk, swing your arms.

THE BOTTOM LINE

Start with an appraisal of your health; give yourself a solid foundation of nutrition, rest, a good mental attitude, and medical care; set attainable, reasonable goals, and you're at the starting line for a physical fitness plan that will work. Whether it's through a structured gymnastic program or via slight changes in behavior throughout the course of your normal day, a combination of aerobic, anaerobic, and flexibility-oriented activities will produce results.

CHAPTER 3

Strong Heart, Strong Body

THE KEYS

• The properly balanced fitness program calls for a well-developed blend of aerobic, anaerobic, and flexibility routines.

• Aerobic training provides an all-body workout to improve cardiovascular health and to reduce body fat, and produces a wide range of physical and emotional benefits.

• Anaerobic, strength, or resistance training is not just for muscle-bound bodybuilders, but important to overall health.

• Be flexible: Limber muscles and tendons plus a good sense of balance and coordination add up to a body that will better profit from any exercise.

• Determining the type, duration, intensity, and frequency of a workout can make the difference between failure and success.

There are three main pieces to a good overall fitness program: aerobic activity to improve cardiovascular endurance and body composition; anaerobic activity to build muscle strength and endurance; and flexibility training to increase your range of motion and lower your risk of injury while you're at work on the other two. Although the aerobics enthusiasts and anaerobics fans often seem to be pulling energetically against each other in a sort of fitness tug-of-war, the fact is you need both.

How Do These Workouts Work?

By understanding how the different approaches do what they do, and what effect they have on your body, you can help your body do them more successfully and with better results. It's much less frustrating to wait for external signs of success when you know progress is taking place inside.

Aerobic

The word *aerobic* literally means "with oxygen." Any activity that causes your heart rate to increase to the point that your body is using oxygen to convert fat and carbohydrates into energy is aerobic (also called cardiovascular, because it calls upon your heart for oxygen pumping and the circulatory system for the oxygen to travel bodywide). Although you reap health benefits from any physical activity, the longer and the more intense the level of exercise, the greater the benefit—as long as you've safely worked up to that level, of course.

Aerobic activity makes your heart stronger, burns fat from all over your body, and boosts your metabolism, making your body a more efficient energy-burning machine. It has been proven to reduce the risks of a long list of diseases—from heart ailments to cancer, immune system disorders to insomnia—and can even better our state of mind. The term *aerobics* for aerobic exercise was coined by Kenneth H. Cooper, M.D., the "Father of Aerobics," of Dallas's Cooper Institute for Aerobics Research.

Anaerobic

Anaerobic simply means "not with oxygen." Anaerobic activity can be separated into two types: movement at a level of exertion below the point at which your body is using oxygen for energy (taking a leisurely stroll, for example, or warming up into an aerobic routine), and exercise of such high intensity (sprinting or lifting heavy objects) that your body requires more energy than aerobic sources can supply. At this point (the anaerobic threshold), the body turns to the muscles for short bursts of power. Although the first type can be credited with refreshing the mind and limbering the muscles, the second is what most people are talking about where physical fitness is concerned.

Anaerobic resistance training, or strength training—using your muscles against various types of weight or opposing force—is the sort of activity that best benefits health. Unlike aerobic training,

SMART SOURCES

American College of
   Sports Medicine
P.O. Box 1440
Indianapolis, IN 46206
800-486-5643
www.acsm.org

The world's largest
sports medicine and
exercise science orga-
nization and, basically,
the last word on
fitness recommenda-
tions of all kinds. The
ACSM Fitness Book
provides illustrated
instruction for aerobic,
resistance and flexi-
bility exercises, along
with fill-in logs and
step-by-step advice on
starting an exercise
routine.

which can be thought of as a bodywide approach to fitness, resistance training works on specific muscles or muscle groups. Traditionally, its health benefits have gone relatively unnoticed. But the American College of Sports Medicine and the American Heart Association, among many others, now recognize the value to such training. Not only does it strengthen, tone, and shape the muscles, but it can prevent and rehabilitate musculoskeletal problems like low-back pain; improve balance, coordination, and agility; and offer all the health benefits associated with leaner body mass (such as reduced risk of various cardiovascular diseases) and improved bone density (lowering the risks of osteoporosis and injury). Whether you're lifting a fifty-pound barbell or the groceries, the stronger your muscles are, the lower the demands on your heart.

Straight for the Heart: Aerobic Training

Depending on how much they jostle you, aerobic activities can be high impact (such as jogging or jumping jacks), which involve heavy contact with a surface; low impact (walking, cycling), which involve moderate impact levels; or no impact (rowing or swimming), which involve fluid, continuous motion. The greater the impact, the greater the stress on your body, which older or more frail exercisers should note.

The Classics

Walking

On the treadmill or on the road, walking is America's most popular form of exercise. A continuing national survey sponsored in part by the Fitness Products Council found it the top choice of frequent exercisers, with 14.5 million of them putting on their walking shoes a hundred times or more in 1996. In the survey's top-ten list of fitness activities, the combined categories of people who fitness-walked and walked on treadmills totaled 65.4 million (with 31.5 million joggers fast on their heels). And in U.S. shopping malls, 3 million people walk for exercise, double the number five years ago, says the National Organization of Mall Walkers. Other than a good pair of shoes, walking requires no special equipment or attire. To get a better workout, add movements to incorporate resistance training and maintain flexibility. Swing your arms, walk uphill, shadowbox, lengthen strides, or carry light weights (in your hands, not around your ankles). Among the features offered by treadmills are varying degrees of incline and movable arm poles, plus all manner of monitors, from speed to mileage.

Cycling

On a stationary cycle or outdoors, cycling provides one of the best cardiovascular workouts, while at the same time strengthening the large muscles of the lower body—including thighs, hips, and buttocks—without putting a lot of stress on the joints. Indoors, some stationary cycles feature movable handles that give your arms a good workout as well. Outdoors, sturdy mountain bikes help navigate rougher roads

F.Y.I.

Top Ten Fitness Activities in 1996 (by millions of participants):

Free weights 42.8

Stationary bicycles 35.0

Treadmills. 32.9

Fitness walking. 32.5

Running/ jogging 31.5

Bicycling. 25.4

Swimming. 23.0

Resistance machines 22.6

Stair-climbing machines 18.2

Step aerobics . . . 11.9

Source: Fitness Products Council

(always wear a helmet), and upper body and arms get into the act when climbing hills. Increase aerobic intensity by shifting into higher gear and pedaling faster, or move into lower gears for a power workout.

In-Line Skating and Skiing

More than 26 million in-line skaters in the United States attest to the enjoyment of this low-impact workout. And skating has a significant impact on fitness levels, especially in the areas of cardiovascular development, lung capacity, muscular strength, and weight loss. Skating is less jarring to your body than running, and just one hour on skates consumes almost as many calories as running and strengthens the muscles and connective tissues surrounding the ankles, knees, and hips. Be sure to wear protective gear: wrist guards, knee and elbow pads, and helmet. Start out slowly on a smooth, flat surface, and increase the level of your workout by skating faster or by skating uphill. Cross-country ski machines (like NordicTrack) simulate the motion of cross-country skiing to exercise the legs and arms.

Jumping Rope

Good, fun, not-just-for-kids stuff that we all know how to do, and that doesn't require a lot of gear. With many cardiovascular benefits, jumping rope improves endurance, and hand and foot coordination as well. Wear comfortable aerobic or cross-training shoes that provide a lot of cushioning for the ball of the foot, and choose a lightweight rope with nonslip foam grips. ("Weighted" ropes or ones with heavy handles can be clumsy.) To find the right length, step one foot on the center of the rope, and bring both handles upward; they should reach about chest high. To add to the workout, try jumping backward, elevate your knees, or get creative with foot patterns.

Swimming and Aquatics

-It's up to fifteen times harder to walk through water than through air, and yet its buoyancy "reduces" your weight by about 90 percent. That translates into more exercise value per movement, and less stress on muscles, bones, and joints. Offered in many class formats, low-impact aquatics, also known as aquasize or aqua aerobics, is a great alternative for those who find the same movements on land too jarring. And exercising in water can greatly improve muscular strength and endurance (the water acts as the resistance) and flexibility (the buoyancy helps joints through a wider range of motion), plus it has cardiovascular and fat-reducing benefits. To increase intensity, enlarge the size of your movement, or increase the speed. For an on-land, water-sport-related workout, try using rowing machines, which work the back, arms, and legs.

Stair Climbing

Taking to the steps instead of the elevator is one of the most readily available exercise options for many city dwellers, and even suburban types can get in on the action on stair-climber machines—continually revolving staircases on which you never quite reach your floor. Good for lower-body toning, with cardiovascular and respiratory benefits, the workout can be performed on StairMaster or other pedal-stepping machines, some of which offer an upper-body workout as well—a sort of pull-up climbing motion to the arms. A cross

F.Y.I.

Who uses what in the weight room (by millions of participants):

Free weights

	1987	1996
Men	17.1	26.0
Women	7.4	16.8

Resistance machines

	1987	1996
Men	8.8	11.1
Women	6.5	11.5

Source: Fitness Products Council

between a stair-climber and a ski machine, elliptical trainers put your legs and feet through a circular, up-and-down motion.

New and Noteworthy

Slide Training

Speed skaters have improvised a version of this for ages, but technology has made this one of the more recently popular exercise activities, performed with a gliding motion on a slick, bumper-edged board about five feet long. While most exercises, like walking and cycling, train your muscles in a forward-and-backward or up-and-down motion, this very-low-impact workout uses the leg and hip muscles involved in sideways movement. Sliding conditions the major muscle groups of the lower body, and the connective tissue between knees, hips, and ankles, targeting hard-to-reach areas of the inner and outer thighs and the buttocks. Because this is an intense activity focusing on seldom-used muscle groups, start off slowly and for short periods of time.

Step/Bench Training

Over the last few years, about 10 million people have used this step-up, step-down, platform method that, when done vigorously, provides the cardiovascular benefits of running with little more stress on the joints than walking would pose. Widely available in a class sessions but easily done at home, step training works on lower-body muscles, and can improve their size and shape. The platform can be adjusted; start at four to six inches (the height should never require bending your knees more than 90 degrees). Change foot patterns to work different sets of muscles, and add arm movements, or raise the step to increase intensity. For advanced steppers only, use propulsion steps, which provide a spring-loaded platform to enhance power moves.

Boxing Aerobics

"The rage around Houston," Dahelia S. Hunt, director of professional fitness instructor training at Texas's Baylor Sports Medicine Institute, calls it. Boxing aerobics is apparently overtaking step training in popularity. Also called cardioboxing, this alternative type of aerobic exercise, a favorite among women as well as men, improves agility, coordination, and balance, along with endurance and strength. With the goal of bettering your fitness rather than rearranging your opponent's nose, you don't have to be Rocky Balboa to reap benefits.

Indoor Cycling

Far from your typical stationary cycle ride, indoor cycling, also known as spinning, studio cycling, and power pacing, among others, is not for the beginner. It was started as a way for road cyclists to train long distances indoors. Standard instructor-led classes average forty minutes, including five minutes or more of warm-up and cool-down. Riders in one study averaged from 75 to 96 percent of their age-predicted heart-rate maximum for most of the class, with most of the participants at the higher end. "Running" (pedaling while standing), "jumping" (coming out of the seat repeatedly while pedaling), and "sprinting" (pedaling furiously for a short time) are just some of the techniques. Most

SMART MONEY

"The best exercises are predicated on your ability to do them," says the International Sports Sciences Association's Charles Staley. "And that depends on physiology as well as skill. Some people are just beating their head into the wall. It's said that squats are 'king of all exercises.' But if you don't have the correct body type, it's not going to work." Get a certified trainer to show you how.

SMART SOURCES

IDEA—International
Association of
Fitness Professionals
6190 Cornerstone Ct. E.
Suite 204
San Diego, CA 92121
800-999-4332
www.ideafit.com

Although not a certi-
fying body, IDEA is one
of the largest member-
ship organizations for
health and fitness
professionals, as well
as a good provider of
exercise and health
lifestyle advice to the
public. A web site
offers fitness tips
including quizzes, news
updates, and fitness
product information
advice, and links to
other reliable sources
for a wide range of
special interest topics.

programs are performed to invigorating music; some guide you along imaginary trails complete with wind, hills, and butterflies; others include choreography such as swaying and upper-body exercise. In all, you sweat like crazy—water bottle and towel are required gear. Padded bike shorts are a good idea. Although indoor cycling is a certified rage at fitness clubs worldwide, research has yet to back up claims about its energy expenditure, adaptability for different fitness levels, and ways to best monitor intensity.

How Long Do You Have to Do It?

The popular thought for many years was that to reap heart-health benefits, you should work out a minimum of twenty minutes, three times a week. Today's research finds three ten-minute sessions just as beneficial to your health.

"If we give a number, people infer that there are no benefits if they don't reach that number. And that's wrong," says Barry Franklin, Ph.D., director of cardiac rehabilitation and exercise laboratories at William Beaumont Hospital in Birmingham, Michigan, and a past vice president of the American College of Sports Medicine. "We're dealing with a time continuum. For the couch potato, eight minutes can be significant. There's nothing magical that occurs between eight and ten minutes, or for that matter between eight and twenty. Rather than a specific frequency, intensity, and duration, it's the total amount of exercise that a person is able to accumulate. And that's a new and key word in exercise science. You can put four quarters or a

Aerobics by Any Other Name . . .

With more and more gyms offering a combination of workout activities, from indoor cycling and martial arts to circuit training and yoga, exercise classes are hardly your father's—or mother's—aerobics anymore.

"Modern workout classes are better and more diversified than ever before—so diversified, in fact, that the term 'aerobics' is no longer an accurate description," says Kathie Davis, executive director of IDEA, an international membership organization of health and fitness professionals. Instead of "aerobics," IDEA recommends that fitness and health promotion industries use the more all-encompassing term "group fitness" instead.

dollar in the piggy bank and ultimately attain the same benefit."

However long you exercise, in order not to undo the good you're trying to gain, warm up and stretch beforehand, then cool down and stretch when you're done (see chapter 2).

Target Zone

A target zone is the place you're aiming to be while you exercise—a level of intensity that can best help your body reach the goals you've set. Working too strenuously can cause injury and exhaustion; working out at too low a level can keep you from reaching your goals. In either case, you'll be discouraged from working out at all.

When exercise people talk about target zones, they're generally referring to staying within a target heart rate (or pulse rate), which is measured in the number of beats per minute (bpm). The zone for the average healthy adult during exercise is generally considered to be between 50 and 85 percent of

"Before I got a heart-rate monitor and I had to measure my pulse myself, I would divide my target heart rate by six," says Haydee Diaz, a twenty-six-year-old receptionist in New York. "That way I could take my pulse for ten seconds and not have to bother with multiplication to figure it out on a per-minute scale."

the average maximum heart rate for people of the same age. Beginners should start at 50 percent of the maximum heart rate (subtract your age from 220 to determine your maximum, then multiply by .50), and work up to 85 percent (subtract your age from 220, then multiply by .85). A forty-year-old, for instance, would do the following math:

220 − 40 = 180 bpm   **(maximum heart rate)**

180 × .50 = 90 bpm   **(lower end of target zone)**

180 × .85 = 153 bpm   **(upper end of target zone)**

Remember, this is an approximation that cardiologists temper with as much as a 20 bpm deviation (a plus-or-minus buffer on either side). Certain medications can affect your maximum heart rate and, in turn, your target zone (consult your doctor to see if this applies to you). The target zone itself can also vary from one exercise to another. For instance, the American Heart Association advises that, because arm exercise produces a higher heart-rate and blood pressure response than does leg exercise, you should lower your target by 10 bpm for exercises involving your arms. In the water, heart rate can be reduced as much as 17 bpm, so if you don't adjust your target zone, you'll think you're not working out hard enough when in actuality you may be overdoing it.

Karvonen Formula

A more personalized method is the Karvonen formula, which takes into account your own heartbeat instead of going by an average-for-your-age heart-rate maximum chart. "The Karvonen method hones in on your fitness level," says Hunt, which can make a big difference in gauging the right level of activity. Figuring out your Karvonen range involves a few more numbers:

1. Find your resting heart rate by taking your pulse first thing in the morning, before you get up and preferably when you've done so without an alarm clock, which can make your heart beat a little faster. Do this for three mornings in a row and record the average.

2. Find your heart-rate reserve (that personal figure) by subtracting your age from 220 and then subtracting your resting heart rate.

3. Multiply your heart-rate reserve by .50 and add back your resting heart rate to get the lower end of your target range.

4. Multiply your heart-rate reserve by .85 and add back your resting heart rate to get the upper end of your target range.

For example, to find the training heart rate of that same forty-year-old, with a resting heart rate of 75 bpm:

$$220 - 40 = 180.00 \text{ bpm} \quad \text{(maximum heart rate)}$$

$$180 - 75 = 105.00 \text{ bpm} \quad \text{(heart-rate reserve)}$$

$$(105 \times .50) + 75 = 127.50 \text{ bpm} \quad \text{(lower end of target zone)}$$

$$(105 \times .85) + 75 = 164.25 \text{ bpm} \quad \text{(upper end of target zone)}$$

Once you know your target zone, you can check that you're within its boundaries in the course of your exercise. Some key times to take your heart rate:

• Before you start: Your heart will be beating faster than the morning resting rate.

• After your warm-up: You'll know that you've warmed up sufficiently if you're nearing the lower end of your target zone.

Variety Workouts

By adding variety to your routine, you can make it more interesting and challenging at the same time as you get a more complete—and safer—body workout. Risks of injury are reduced when the same muscles, bones, and joints aren't subjected to the stresses of the same activity over and over again. Performance improves, and it makes it easier to increase exercise intensity without burning out.

Take your choice: Keep it all aerobic, all resistance, or mix it up on different days or within the same session. Work on single muscles or on groups; change your pace, the time spent on each activity, and the rest periods in between—whatever works for you.

• **Circuit training.** Great for the person with a limited amount of time per workout, circuit training involves a continuous change of activity: five minutes on the treadmill, ten reps of free weights, ten minutes on the stationary cycle, and so on. Circuit weight training combines light- to moderate-intensity weight training with aerobic activity by keeping you moving between ten to fifteen stations (the individual pieces of equipment) with little rest (fifteen to thirty seconds) in between. You shouldn't lift as much weight as you would in the traditional weight-training routine, but by increasing the number of reps and staying continually active, the muscles work just as hard.

• During your routine: Just be sure that you don't stop cold to do it, which could strain your heart.

• After you've cooled down: Your heart should be close to the pre-exercise rate.

Remember, the benefits of a good aerobic exercise program include a slower heartbeat, so if you're following the Karvonen formula, check your resting heart rate every few weeks, and update your target zone. Keep track of the

Circuit training increases maximum oxygen uptake in a way that traditional weight training (with more than one to two minutes' rest between sets) can't. Other benefits: reduced burn, and less chance of overstressing muscles, tendons, and ligaments. But remember not to rush—take time to properly adjust every apparatus before you use it.

• **Interval training.** This method alternates short bursts of intense activity with active recovery, which is just a less intense version of the same thing.

Fartlek is one form of interval training. The less-than-elegant Swedish term translates into "run play" or "speed play," and usually refers to adding intervals of slow trotting or running to a walking routine. You might jog to the nearest mailbox, for the duration of a snappy song on your headset, or just as long as you feel comfortable. Unlike traditional interval training, fartlek doesn't involve preset periods of time or levels of intensity; how you feel determines the activity and the intensity.

• **Cross training.** Cross training involves varying your routine from workout to workout, or within the same session. You might play tennis on Monday, lift free weights on Wednesday, jump rope on Friday, and work out on the Nautilus machine over the weekend. Or, in a less intense form of circuit training, alternate within a single workout, with fifteen minutes on the treadmill, say, and fifteen minutes using an exercise band. Jog to the pool, swim, and walk home. You could also switch between low- and high-impact aerobics, or activities that target different muscle groups, like slide training and lat pull-downs.

changes in your personal log, and take pride in your progress: The four-miles-per-hour pace that had you huffing and puffing at 70 percent levels

How to Take Your Pulse

Manually:

Gently touch the two first fingers (not your thumb) of one hand to the pulse point at the base of the thumb (radial artery) on the other hand, or to the carotid artery, at the side of the neck. Do not press too hard because this can actually slow down the flow of blood. Count the number of beats in a ten-second period, and multiply by six for your beats per minute (bpm).

With a Heart-Rate Monitor:

To eliminate some of the work from your workout, use an electronic heart-rate monitor—there are versions available to suit everybody. Most sense cardiac activity with electrodes in a chest-strap transmitter that sends the information to a wrist-watch display; some use photocell or infrared sensors to do the job. As for accuracy, a study that compared the devices with $20,000 electrocardiogram (ECG) machines found many to be "ECG accurate"—within six beats per minute of the ECG 95 percent of the time.

Some have built-in interference blockers to eliminate confusing signals from the heart-rate monitor of the person working out next to you; others offer computer interface systems; others will beep when you stray outside your target zone. One of the newest models on the market, the HEARTalker by New Life Technologies, provides 250 prerecorded "motivational" messages featuring the voice of a TV fitness host (and a mute button, too).

Price is a reflection of the number of features, not accuracy: The $429 Polar Cyclovantage was one of twenty-eight popular models found ECG-accurate in a *ConsumerMatters* (American Council on Exercise) report. So was the $79 Acumen Target-Trac.

Although your best bet is a monitor that is attached to you rather than the machine on which you're working, none are perfect. Use them simply as helpful guides.

in the beginning might soon be a comfortable, easy 50 percent.

A Better Way

If you're not crazy about math—or sketchy approximations—you're in good company. More and more health professionals are abandoning the heartbeat counting for another method.

"They're just too tabular," says Gerald Fletcher, M.D., a cardiologist at Mayo Clinic Jacksonville and professor of medicine at the Mayo Medical School, about the inaccuracy of estimated maximum heart-rate scales. "The only real safe, accurate way is to have an exercise test in the presence of a health professional." And even then, following estimated heart-rate zones can deceive.

Fletcher, Hunt, and many others are encouraging exercisers to use a rate-perceived exertion (RPE) scale, a personal assessment of your workout that takes into account not only your heartbeat but other metabolic processes as well (see chapter 2). Even with a perfectly calculated maximum heart rate, your body may react to exercise in an unpredictable way. With the RPE method, you assign a number (say, 0 to 10, with 10 measuring maximum exertion) to the way your body feels throughout your workout. The recommended RPE range for most people during exercise is between 3 (moderate) and 5 (strong); you decide for yourself what level of activity rates a 3 and what rates a 5 for you. Also known as the Borg Rating of Perceived Exertion, it uses a scale of 6 to 20 as well. (Don't ask us why.)

"Talk tests" are another valuable measure: If you can talk while you're exercising, you're not overdoing it.

Exercise Caution: Signs That You're Overdoing It

- Decreased performance
- Longer recovery time
- Headache
- Muscle soreness
- Decreased ability to resist infection

- Loss of coordination
- Higher resting heart rate
- Loss of appetite
- Stomachache
- Dizziness

One of the most common mistakes of the enthusiastic new exerciser is doing too much, too fast, or for too long a period of time. Sometimes the motivation is to get it over with. In other cases, workouts become an addiction, a substitute for other parts of life. Exercising beyond the point of exhaustion, while injured, or to the exclusion of the many other aspects of a healthy existence are warning signs. Overuse syndrome, a tendency to exercise excessively, puts you at risk not only of poor performance, but injury and unhappiness. And that's not what fitness is about.

"Just go to the point where it's hard, where you're sweating a little bit, having a little trouble talking," says Fletcher. "That is the best guideline. The RPE is being used more and more so [target calculations don't] become too much of a science, to the point where people are working with gimmickry rather than going ahead and exercising."

Healthy Strength: Resistance Training

How do you measure strength fitness? "Strength fitness means that your muscles are strong enough for you to do not only the activities of daily life, but recreational activities, and most of the other things that people want to accomplish, comfortably," says Daniel Kosich, Ph.D., president of Exerfit Consulting in Denver and a consultant to the IDEA-International Association of Fitness Professionals in San Diego. "While there are fairly definitive measurements of aerobic fitness, there's no real demarcation line in terms of strength between fit and not fit."

A good resistance-training routine will take into account your fitness goals and abilities, and address all your body's muscle groups. Train on a weekly cycle, working different muscles at each session. There are a lot of options: slow or fast tempo; short or long rest periods; the number of times you do the exercises, and what kind and how many you do; and whether you use weights or not. The range of approaches can easily make your head spin, and has been the source of much debate. And, as with any exercise program, resistance-training routines need to be varied in order to prevent boredom and injury, and accommodate higher levels of fitness as you progress.

Charles Staley, B.Sc., M.S.S., director of program development at the International Sports Sciences Association in Santa Barbara, California, an Olympic weightlifting coach, and founder of Myo Dynamics, a consulting firm, confirms this fact: "Every day I talk to people who have been at a plateau in their training for months or even years, usually due to long-term overreliance on one limited method of training."

Abs

Rectus abdominis. Just under the chest down to a few inches below the naval.

Bis

Biceps. Two muscles at the front of the upper arm.

Delts

Deltoids. Shoulders; the muscles around the tops of the arms.

Glutes

Gluteus maximus. The "buns"; the largest muscles in the body.

Hams

Hamstrings. The three muscles at the back of each thigh.

Resistance-Training Activities

Whether you're working with the weight of a physical object (be it a barbell or a soup can), against the tension of stretchable exercise bands, or against the pull of gravity on your own body (leg lifts and curl-ups), the proper resistance-training program takes into account your fitness requirements, including strength, flexibility, and stamina, in a way that doesn't overemphasize any one muscle group. One day's workout might focus on legs, buttocks, and midsection; another might center on back, shoulders, arms, and chest.

Major Muscle Groups

• Shoulders: Deltoids, rotator cuff

• Arms: Biceps, triceps, forearm muscles

• Chest: Pectorals

• Back (upper): Trapezius

• Back (midsection and lower): Latissimus dorsi, lumbar (spinal) erectors

• Legs (upper): Quadriceps, hamstrings, adductors, hip flexors

• Legs (lower): Gastrocnemius, soleus

• Buttocks/hips: Gluteus maximus, gluteus medius

• Midsection: Abdominals, obliques

Invest in a simple anatomy chart or photocopy a chart from a book in the library to find out where these muscles are.

As for exercises, there are dozens. Abdominal curl-ups or workouts on a back-extension machine strengthen abdominal and back muscles, improving strength and posture. Floor or machine crunches can work the stomach muscles; wrist curls strengthen the forearms; heel raises tone the calves. There are push-ups, pull-ups, and sit-ups, lunges and dips. And these are a limited sampling, to be sure.

Which exercises are the "right" ones? "The best exercises are the ones you're going to do," says Kosich. "There are lots of good ways to get strong—push-ups, sit-ups, ab and lower-back exercises—that don't require any weights."

Check with a certified fitness professional to learn which exercises are appropriate, and the safe and effective technique involved. Otherwise you can hurt yourself. Seated leg extensions can damage the cartilage on the underside of the kneecap, for instance. Although squats can strengthen the thighs, they can also injure your back.

How you do the exercise is key. "Subtleties of exercise performance are the thing," says Charles Staley. "It can't be stressed enough how nuance of performance can take you from an exercise doing nothing to that same exercise doing everything."

How Long Do You Have to Do It?

Resistance-training exercises of all kinds are measured in the number of repetitions (or reps),

SMART DEFINITIONS

Lats
Latissimus dorsi. The largest back muscle, from the lower back to below the shoulders.

Pecs
Pectorals. The chest muscles.

Quads
Quadriceps. The four muscles at the front of each thigh.

Traps
Trapezius. The back muscle that extends from the neck to the shoulders and down to the center of the back.

Tris
Triceps. The back of the upper arms.

meaning the number of times you perform each exercise, and in sets, a group of repetitions performed at a time. A high number of repetitions using lower amounts of resistance (the weight or force against which you push or pull) encourages the development of speed, flexibility, and stamina; fewer repetitions with heavier resistance encourages strength, size, and power.

The speed with which you see results—why some people increase in muscle size and others don't—has to do with genetics and body type. Muscular mesomorphs, for example, respond to strength training by building muscle mass much faster than slim ectomorphs, even with the same training regime. Curvy endomorphs generally need to lose body fat to see any change in muscle size or shape.

Exercisers interested in bodybuilding may do multiple sets of any one exercise, but for health benefits, the American College of Sports Medicine, the American Heart Association, and the Surgeon General's Report on Physical Activity and Health recommend that people under the age of fifty perform one set of eight to ten different exercises, with eight to twelve reps of each, two to three times per week, with at least forty-eight hours' rest in between. Those over fifty should follow the same regimen, but with ten to fifteen reps instead of eight to twelve. (That doesn't mean that people over fifty are working out harder, but at lighter levels of resistance that won't tax older cardiovascular systems, bones, ligaments, and joints.)

Start with the amount of weight that allows you to do eight or ten reps in good form and with good technique—not so little that you could do another eight hundred easily, but just enough so that by number eight or ten, you're glad you're done.

When that gets easier, move to the higher number of reps, and when you can do those correctly, without getting overly tired, increase the amount of resistance and start back at the lower rep point.

Says Daniel Kosich, "The eight-to-twelve range takes away the uncertainty of across-the-board weight recommendations that don't at all take into account the differences between the capabilities of a ninety-pound woman and a two-hundred-pound man."

Resistance Equipment: The Classics

When you're shopping for a house, the three most important things are location, location, location. With exercise, it's technique, technique, technique. Not even the best piece of equipment will do any good if handled incorrectly, and may cause physical harm. Contact a local gym or certified trainer for individual or class sessions (for advice on finding a good personal trainer, see chapter 4).

Free Weights

Barbells or dumbbells are the basics. A barbell is the larger, heavier piece of equipment, with a fixed or changeable weight. Dumbbells are shorter, smaller versions of barbells that are lifted with one hand.

Multi-Station Machines

These are the home gyms so often hawked on infomercials. They usually are based on a system of elastic resistance or have cables attached to weights or flexible poles. Features offer workouts

SMART DEFINITIONS

Burn
The feeling in a muscle that has been worked intensely.

Cut Up/Ripped
A lean body or muscle with highly visible muscle contour.

Definition
The quality of being cut up, or ripped.

Pumped
Temporarily swelled, as happens to muscles after exercise.

Sticking Point
A normal plateau that occurs when a muscle resists enlargement, no matter how hard it's worked.

on several muscle groups, with adjustable settings for positioning and weight.

Exercise Tubing and Bands

Under the umbrella term "rubber-resistive products," these stretchy tubes and bands allow resistance movements that are difficult to accomplish with other strength-training devices and, with proper technique and positioning, can be a valuable workout tool for beginners and experienced lifters alike. Portable and inexpensive, they're also good complements to conventional free-weight training, since the lighter resistance helps prefatigue the muscle during warm-up exercise. (But they're not limited to easy lifts: The Flexband can simulate loads from one to a thousand pounds of pressure when several bands are used in combination.) Special sports-specific attachments are available for golf, baseball, and tennis training.

Stability Ball

Sold under the name Physio Ball, Resist-A-Ball, and others, these colorful, extra-large, inflatable vinyl balls are designed to improve balance and develop the often-neglected abdomen, chest, and back muscles that stabilize the rest of the body. Performing exercises on the ball challenges muscles to maintain alignment, which helps build postural endurance and synchronicity of movement. Studies have also found that people exercising on the ball gained cardiovascular benefits not attained by those exercising on a seat. Peanut-shaped stability balls are available for those with severe balance or mobility problems.

New and Noteworthy

Pilates, or the Method

Don't let the Reformer, a wooden apparatus with cables, pulleys, springs, and sliding boards, scare you away. The Pilates (pronounced puh-LAH-teez) Method that uses it offers a mind-body approach to fitness that focuses on improving total body flexibility and strength without build-

Women and Weights

The number of women who exercised with free weights more than doubled to 16.8 million in 1996, from 7.4 million in 1987, according to the Fitness Products Council. On resistance machines, women outnumber men. The number of women who use them has increased 75 percent since 1987, to 11.5 million from 6.5 million (11.1 million men use the machines).

The benefits of weight training for women are clear. And while many used to avoid resistance training for fear of looking like Hulk Hogan, more and more are realizing that the health benefits, including important increases in bone density, outweigh the almost negligible risks of becoming unwillingly muscle-bound.

Women may have less of the muscle-building testosterone hormone in their systems, but they need resistance training just as much as men do. "Between the genders, the importance of muscle strength is equal," says Daniel Kosich, Ph.D. "Because women have a more substantial risk for osteoporosis, strength training adds a more valuable component. Strength training is one of the best ways to decrease the risk."

Women should follow a general major muscle program, with special attention to upper body and upper back, common areas of weakness. And those who wear high heels are prone to shortened calf muscles and tendons, so that area may need to be addressed. Working with a qualified trainer to develop a balanced strength-training program is crucial.

What Matters

• Proper technique and posture while exercising.

• Warming up and cooling down before and after every exercise.

• Staying in touch with your level of exertion.

• A balanced program of aerobic, resistance, and flexibility exercise.

• Recovery time between resistance exercises.

What Doesn't

• What particular method you use.

• Popular but inaccurate fitness myths.

• Looking like Mr. or Ms. Universe.

• Sticking to one and only one routine.

• Ego.

ing bulk. "Not just exercise," the Pilates Studio would say. The series of controlled movements performed on specifically designed equipment and offered in small groups was developed by Joseph H. Pilates seventy years ago. Martha Graham and George Balanchine were among the first of many dancers to use it; today Hollywood celebs have popularized the non-impact technique. The focus is on the abdominal and back muscles—referred to as the body's core—in a routine of a very few but extremely precise repetitions in several planes of motion, and on breathing patterns that don't always follow the exhale-on-exertion pattern of traditional exercise. Trademark issues have some studios calling their Pilates-like technique "the Method," "the Physicalmind Workout," or even "the P Word." Floor-work classes are available as well.

Plyometrics

Also known as jump training, this technique involves leaping from boxes or benches on the theory that stretching the muscles before contracting them will strengthen muscles, increase vertical jump, and decrease impact forces on the joints. Participants in a combined program of stretching, plyometric training, and weight training increased their hamstring strength by 44 percent, and studies have found it to have a positive effect on bone density in younger participants. Beginners may start off by jumping over cones or foam barriers, gradually increasing to more difficult exercises (at the more radical end, "depth jumping" or "drop jumping" has involved forty-two-inch leaps), but plyometrics is not for anyone in poor shape. Using a coach or trainer can make this program safe and effective, but athletic prowess, not fitness, is the emphasis here. Fitness-seekers may not find the risks worth taking.

Safe Training That Works

Studies have shown that even ninety-year-olds can benefit from a good strength-training program, so don't let the image of greased-up bodybuilders with Schwarzeneggeresque physiques kick sand in the face of your fitness goals. Follow a sensible routine, keeping in mind the following advice, and you'll have a fitter body and better health.

• **Warm up.** Stretches and a low-resistance set of exercises are good ways to rehearse the muscles you're going to use in your routine.

• **Employ proper technique.** Work out in a slow, rhythmic manner, at a full range of motion. Repetitions should be about four seconds: Raise the weight for a count of two; lower it for a count of two. Although there may be some power benefits to a longer release (or negative phase), the two-two count is easy and less taxing to your body. Full range of motion involves moving the part of the body you're exercising as far as possible.

• **Balance your workouts.** If you don't balance your workouts to address all the muscle groups, with more emphasis on weak areas to bring them up to speed, you risk muscle size and strength imbalances, as well as injury, postural problems, and other musculoskeletal ills. Stability training refers to learning proper body balance to work out with better technique.

• **Work at your own level.** Pay attention to how your body feels during as well as after a workout, and use common sense. If you're in pain or cannot function the morning after, you're doing too much or doing it the wrong way. And if you stop for a few weeks, don't start up again right where you were; build up gradually.

• **Don't push progression.** Progression—systematically increasing the stress a muscle endures during an exercise—cannot be rushed. Whether you progress by increasing the weight, by increasing the number of repetitions, by increasing the number of sets, or by decreasing the amount of rest between sets, do it gradually.

• **Allow recovery time.** To avoid burnout and injury, allow at least forty-eight hours between exercises of any muscle or muscle group.

• **Work with a qualified instructor.** Not even the most thorough fitness book or video can substitute for a certified personal trainer in teaching proper technique. "People think that they can go up to a piece of equipment and they're safe," says Dahelia Hunt. "Most people haven't been taught how to move the equipment, rather than having the equipment move them."

• **Get started.** Don't let the fear of a lengthy contracts or long-term commitment to a trainer put you off. One to three sessions will be worth more than their weight in fitness and health.

THE BOTTOM LINE

If you want to be physically fit, aerobic and resistance training join flexibility exercises as essential parts of the plan. Too often we are discouraged by false notions about what that means we have to do. The truth is, we can do it most any way we like best—whether that means walking on a treadmill at a gym or taking a tour of the neighborhood; lifting barbells or doing floor exercise. The only thing that matters is that we do it sensibly, with a balanced, personal program that suits our needs.

CHAPTER 4

....

Joining a Gym

Almost 21 million people belong to the more than 13,000 commercial health clubs in the United States, reports the International Health, Racquet and Sportsclub Association (IHRSA) in Boston. That's more than twice as many clubs as existed in 1987, but only half as many as IHRSA expects to be around by 2010.

Last year, health clubs, gyms, sports clubs, wellness centers—there is no one politically correct term—contributed an estimated $8.5 billion to the nation's GNP. Someone's paying more than attention out there.

Why Go to a Gym?

When in Rome, you do as the Romans; when in a gym, you exercise. And while it might not be Exercise Eden for everybody (we'll explore the alternatives in chapter 5), the energetic hustle-and-bustle of the health club or gym can provide a motivating backdrop to your own fitness activity.

Beyond a variety of state-of-the-art equipment that offers a plethora of choice (try affording it, much less storing it in that extra room), gyms have professionals to help you, classes to inspire you, safeguards to protect you, supportive fellow exercisers to encourage you, and a surefire way to keep you off the couch (it's at home; you're not).

If you enjoy a partner sport like racquetball or a team sport like basketball, you'll find others of similar stripe. If you're surrounded by fitness options, there's a greater chance of trying something new: While you're working out on the treadmill, you might start thinking the step class looks like fun.

You take a momentary break on the La-Z-Boy-lookalike leg-press machine, and someone offers to teach you a new resistance-training exercise.

Some offer healthy lifestyle programs—nutrition, smoking cessation, or stress management—to help you in wide-ranging areas of health. Others offer child care to put your mind at ease.

Gyms can help you with a solid fitness foundation in more ways than one, with injury-reducing, effectiveness-improving surfaces on which to work out. While it's safe to do low- to moderate-impact aerobics on the living room carpet, for instance, it's not a proper surface for high-impact routines. For basketball, indoor wood courts are much safer than outdoor asphalt or concrete.

Last but hardly least, if you're the kind of person who needs to make an external sign of his or her commitment to fitness, joining a gym can mean you mean business when you say you mean to get fit. Think of it as making an appointment with better health.

Why Do Most Gym-Goers Go?

For women of all ages, the primary reason is weight control, according to an IHRSA survey, with toning muscles in second place among those age eighteen to thirty-four, and cardiovascular conditioning for women thirty-five and up. Men's primary motivation changes with age: strength training for eighteen- to twenty-four-year-olds (followed by weight control) and weight control for those twenty-five to fifty-four (with health concerns becoming increasing important with age). For those fifty-five and over, cardiovascular training is number one, with weight control second on the list.

Health Club Membership

Women

Number: 11,823,000
Percentage of club
membership: 56.7%
Change from 1987: ....up 64%
Average visits to the
club per year: 82

Men

Number: 9,010,000
Percentage of club
membership: ....43.3 %
Change from 1987: ....up 37%
Average visits to the
club per year: 88

Source: International Health, Racquet and
Sportsclub Association, 1996

Who uses the club most? Not the youngsters. Men age sixty-five and over are the leaders, averaging 139 days a year, followed by men age forty-five to fifty-four (114) and women age sixty-five and over (108). Membership doesn't mean usership, either: While almost 57 percent of club members are women, men tend to visit the club more often; although those with annual incomes of $75,000 or greater make up one third of the members, and those with under $25,000 account for 16 percent, the latter group uses the club far more often (84 versus 112 days a year).

Choosing the Right Gym

If you find the presence of other exercisers more intimidating than inspiring, or just would rather do your workouts far from the hum of machines and the occasional grunt from a lifter, a fitness club might not be the right place for you. But if you're one of the many who can draw on that energy, you've got more than 13,000 choices available. Here's how to narrow that down.

Location

The most important criteria in choosing? "Convenience," says Cathy Masterson McNeil, of IHRSA.

"It has to be close to where you work or where you live. Most people will not travel more than five miles by car, or ten minutes if they have to walk to it. And especially when people are just starting an exercise program, they'll think of reasons not to go. 'It's raining.' 'There's no time to get there.' You just have to remove that obstacle."

People

Are employees and instructors experienced, supportive, and friendly? Are trainers certified by nationally recognized certifying agencies (see "Personal Trainers: Do You Need One?" on page 80) and do they have educational backgrounds in the health and fitness field? Are they trained in cardiopulmonary resuscitation (CPR)? Will they willingly provide new members with a club orientation and instruction on how to use equipment? Will they check on, and record, your progress as you go along? If you're not comfortable with the staff of the facility, or can't trust them to give you helpful advice, you'll be less likely to want to be around them and to get the instruction for which you've signed on.

The membership can make a difference, too. Are you there to meet people or learn from them? Does it bother or inspire you to exercise in a crowd? Will you be surrounded by he-man bodybuilders or working-out moms interested

Nationally Recognized Certifying Agencies

• Aerobics and Fitness Association of America

• American Aerobics Association/International Sports Medicine Association

• American College of Sports Medicine

• American Council on Exercise

• Cooper Institute for Aerobics Research

• National Academy of Sports Medicine

• National Association for Fitness Certification

• National Federation of Professional Trainers

• National Strength and Conditioning Association

There are numerous certifying bodies in addition to those listed above, many focusing on specific fitness fields. Be sure to check credentials thoroughly.

Red Flags

• No fitness evaluation or health-screening routines.

• Complaints against the facility filed with the Better Business Bureau or other local consumer protection agency.

• Offers of prepaid, lifetime memberships (illegal in most states).

• Hard-sell salespeople and pushy tactics.

• Resistance to let you speak with members privately or see all areas of the club.

• Reluctance to provide you with written information about your agreement and rights.

in taking off a few pounds? The people you see at the gym can tell you a lot about its orientation, and affect your comfort level during your own workout as well.

Facility and Equipment

Is the facility clean, well-maintained, and well-ventilated? Is lighting sufficient, and are noise levels comfortable? Is the equipment in good shape, or labeled if it's broken? Is there enough of it to offer you a sufficient variety of workout options, and accommodate the number of people there when you're going to work out? Are signs posted near the equipment to remind you how it should be used? Is the flooring kept smooth and dry? Are lockers provided? Are pools, whirlpools, and saunas sparkling? Are workout areas in good condition? An establishment that can't keep itself in good shape isn't likely to be able to help you.

Activities and Services

You might start out just wanting to flex those biceps and pedal a mile or two on the stationary cycle, but as you get into the habit of bettering your body, your horizons will likely expand. Does the club offer a variety of programs to broaden your scope? Classes in step training, yoga, swimming, stress management, smoking cessation? Are there qualified instructors to lead them? Convenient times to take them? Will the club provide you with child care if you need it? Or recreational off-site social activities?

Cost

IHRSA estimates most people pay between $300 and $600 for a year's membership, with the average closer to $325. Clubs with spas, salons, and other upscale offerings—from car detailing to travel agencies on-site—can run higher, up to $1,000 and well beyond. And then there are those like the super-luxe Houstonian Club, where monthly Resident Membership dues, including complete dining, social, and athletic use of the club, are $186—after a $14,000 initiation fee. (More on the Houstonian in chapter 8.)

Longer-term agreements usually cost less overall than a month-to-month contract, but might not be worth it if you're not sure you'll be in the area for an extended period of time. You'll often find that you can negotiate a better deal for yourself if you just ask. If a friend is already paying less at that club due to a previous special offer, or you've been extended better rates at another place, salespeople may be agreeable to meeting or beating that price. Worth a try.

For Safety's Sake

Whether you're looking for the world's most basic health club or one with all the whistles and bells, user safety is an absolute must. Not only must the

F.Y.I.

Amount spent by Americans on sports shoes in the first six months of 1997: More than $6.5 billion.

Source: Sporting Goods Manufacturers Association

physical plant and its surroundings be free of structural hazards, but your planned program of activity must be clear of any hazards itself. Is a health history questionnaire, fitness test, and health evaluation properly taken to see if a doctor's input is needed before you start? Is the club equipped with a fully stocked, accessible first-aid kit? Does the facility have liability insurance?

Chain or Independent?

The larger gyms, like Bally's or Gold's Gym, with multiple locations, may allow you to take advantage of their other facilities, which is helpful if you travel a lot or relocate. Because they have a large number of employees and members, the chances of class cancellations are lower; membership rates tend to be less expensive; and more programs might be offered than at independent gyms. On the down side, if you're not one who wants to blend in with the crowd, you'll probably mind that being one person among so many lessens the odds of personalized attention from a sometimes harried staff.

Some Hints

No brochure can provide the answers to the many things you need to know before signing up with a gym. For that, you need a personal tour or, better yet, a trial visit. Not only will you learn what the place looks, sounds, feels, and smells like, but it will give you a good idea of the attentiveness level you'll be able to expect from the staff.

Be sure to schedule your tour or visit at a time

when you plan to be there for your workout—the calm and spacious facility you see at two in the afternoon on a weekday might be a different story altogether when you show up for your after-work routine. Take the time to talk to a few clients in private for some unbiased opinions of the club's weak points and strengths.

Talk to friends and coworkers to see if they can make any recommendations (or extend a free guest pass for you to give it a try), and visit a few places before deciding on one. Remember, the better your understanding of your fitness goals, the better you'll be able to find a place that can meet them.

Before Signing on the Dotted Line

What does exercise have in common with reading contracts? Everyone knows it's good for you, but many of us don't do it. Before you become a member of a club, it's important to check the contract to be sure you know what you're signing up for, how long you're signing up for it, and how much it's really going to cost.

• **Double-check verbal agreements.** Check to see that any verbal agreements or offers are in writing. If the special deal you're being extended isn't spelled out in the contract, have the salesperson write it out and initial the additional details.

• **Understand the length of the contract.** There are many types: multi-year, annual, several months at a time, or month-to-month. Prepaid lifetime memberships are a definite no-no, illegal in most states.

SMART MONEY

Whether to go to a gym or work out at home? "Don't think of it as an either/or situation," says Cathy Masterson McNeil, of IHRSA. While club membership can provide many starting exercisers with the boost they need to get into a regular exercise habit, there will be times when you can't get there. "Take a walk, ride a bike," McNeil advises. There's no need to confine your health to the health club.

SMART SOURCES

Consult these organizations for help in finding a certified trainer:

Aerobics and Fitness
    Association of
    America
800-225-2322
www.afaa.com

American College of
    Sports Medicine
800-486-5643
www.acsm.org

American Council on
    Exercise
800-529-8227
www.acefitness.org

National Federation of
    Professional Trainers
800-729-6378
www.nfpt.com

• **Look for an out.** We're not encouraging you to go back to the sofa, but do find out about whether there's a cooling-off period to protect you from overzealous salespeople and their ploys; many state laws allow you up to three days after signing to cancel the agreement without penalty. You may also want to check to see what other cancellation provisions are in the contract in case you become disabled or move away. Some clubs will extend your contract if you have to leave town for extended business trips or if you're incapacitated for a length of time.

• **Check ownership.** Will the club "own" your contract? Or will they sell it to a third party, and so have less of a stake in your continuing satisfaction?

• **Be aware of your rights.** Many states regulate contract length and cancellation policies. Call your local consumer protection agency or attorney general's office to find out about yours.

Personal Trainers: Do You Need One?

Just because you're not Oprah Winfrey doesn't mean you can't afford a personal trainer. Or benefit from one. Whether you're looking for occasional help at the gym, a pull-you-out-of-bed visit every morning, or anything in between, a qualified trainer can be a big help in the success of your fitness regime.

Coach, teacher, role model, motivator, confidant—these are just a few of the roles a personal trainer plays. A good, personal-tailored, trainer-designed program based on a professional evaluation of your fitness level stands a better chance of getting you where you want to be. A trainer can help you establish realistic short- and long-term goals and a plan of action, then work with you to set a schedule that suits your needs: frequent, ongoing visits to keep you accountable, or a few appointments to familiarize you with your workout, followed by a scheduled checkup and reevaluation a few weeks down the road.

Many people use trainers when they're recover-

The Perfect Gym Bag:
What You Need and How to Pack It

Some gyms provide towels, hair blowers, self-locking lockers, even shampoo. Others don't. Pack accordingly.

- Membership card

- Water bottle

- Comfortable workout clothes (loose enough to allow flexibility, but not so loose that they'll get caught in machinery or get in your way)

- Appropriate shoes for each activity, and socks

- Sweatband and/or hair tie

- Weight-lifting gloves

- Towels (to take with you during your workout, and for the shower)

- Plastic bag for dirty clothes

- Toiletries (soap, shampoo, deodorant, brush or comb)

- Shower sandals

- Locker lock

- Portable radio or cassette headset, and extra batteries

- Reading material

- Heart-rate monitor

- Fresh clothing to wear home (especially if you're coming from work and don't want to put your suit back on)

Gym Do's and Don'ts

Do

• Clean up after yourself: Wipe down benches and equipment when you're done.

• Put equipment back where it belongs.

• Dress reasonably: Don't force people to see more of your body than they want.

• Share (do not hog) the equipment: If you'll be long, let someone work in a set.

• Ask for help from staff, not other clients.

• Keep the grunting noises to yourself.

• Wash, and use liberal amounts of deodorant.

Don't

• Leave your gym bag or other possessions where others can trip over them.

• Spit in the water fountain.

• "Jawsercise": A gym's no place to work out your mouth.

• Sing out loud to your headphones.

• Stay naked in the locker room, no matter how great your physique.

• Let someone get hurt: Alert an instructor and let him/her provide the help.

• Laugh at anyone else's technique or physique.

• Wear perfume or cologne.

ing from physical injury, or to help them prepare for a special athletic event. Others count on them for their knowledge of up-to-date fitness information and research. But it's the help they provide in your fight to stay motivated—the greatest battle of all—that you'll hear being praised over and over. The mere existence of your appointment can keep you from "I'll do it tomorrow" thoughts, and their encouragement and expertise can help them push you just enough to expand your body's capabilities, without causing harm.

"Most people make the mistake of doing too

much too soon, and end up not feeling good, or their muscles hurt, or they don't have a good time and so they quit," says Pam Germain, M.S., of the National Association for Fitness Certification (NAFC). "When I ease them into their program, they usually end up sticking to it because it does not hurt as much. A good certified personal trainer will treat them in a way that helps them to gradually progress."

Finding the Right Trainer

In choosing a trainer, determine whether you'll be working with one at the gym you belong to or at your home. Many have a facility of their own to offer; if so, evaluate it—from convenience to equipment—on the same criteria you would use when choosing a health club or gym.

Many of the same things you look for in a gym are desirable in a trainer as well. Both should offer a pleasant—as well as healthful and educational—experience. Both should take your personal health requirements into account, and be able to offer you experience and good references. Both should be able to provide a convenient schedule at a price you can afford, with understandable written contracts that outline your agreement, including cancellation policies, billing, and any "exceptional" fees. Both should have liability insurance. Both need to give you what you need.

The American Council on Exercise certified 6,454 trainers in 1996, and IDEA, the membership association of fitness professionals, estimates the number of certified trainers nationwide at more than 55,000.

F.Y.I.

The Nike Swoosh represents the wing of the Greek goddess after whom the company was named. Its designer, Caroline Davidson, was a student at Portland State University in 1971 when Phil Knight (today Nike's Chairman of the Board and CEO), who was teaching accounting classes at the school, asked her to design a logo that could be placed on the side of a shoe.

"She handed him the Swoosh," Nike historians tell us. "He handed her thirty-five dollars.

Nike's total revenues for the second quarter of fiscal year 1998: $2.26 billion.

STREET SMARTS

"She has me doing things I never would have thought possible," says Louis Turner, a forty-three-year-old health professional, of his circuit-training sessions with a personal trainer. A former fitness club user who found himself more and more reluctant to make it to the gym, he's been working out three times a week without fail. "Without her, I just wouldn't do it."

Look for Certification

To design a safe, effective workout, a trainer should have a good knowledge of everything from exercise physiology and injury prevention to motivational techniques, with the proof in certification through a nationally recognized organization (most require recertification every two to four years) and, if possible, a degree in a related medical or physical science field.

Many consider the American College of Sports Medicine certification program to be the gold standard, with written and practical exams in applying scientific principles of conditioning and motivational techniques for establishing a healthy, overall lifestyle. Among the many other qualifications for which ACSM looks in a trainer are work-related experience, or educational degrees; skill in the many methods of fitness appraisal; ability to evaluate the physical and emotional effects of regular exercise, and to improve them; ability to teach lifestyle modification; and current CPR certification.

Like many certifying groups, ACSM offers different certification levels. Health/Fitness Instructor is appropriate for personal trainers, while Exercise Leader certification is geared to those who'll be at the head of an exercise class. Other certifications might focus on aerobics, or weight loss, or strength and conditioning specialties. Find a trainer with training applicable to what you want to do. And if you need to question the organization's credentials, you might want to continue your search.

Other Qualifications

There are many important things to consider in choosing a trainer that go beyond that certificate on the wall. Is he a good teacher? A good listener? Someone who bypasses fitness jargon for words you'll understand? Does she take the time to find out who you are—in terms of personality as well as pec size—and what you want to accomplish, or put you through his "signature" routine? Will he offer the drill sergeant discipline you're seeking, or do you want a more gentle, encouraging approach? Does she have an agreement with any one equipment manufacturer or store? If so, is it a reputable firm, or are commercial interests going to supersede good product recommendations and advice?

Does she give you her full attention the whole session, or get distracted by others, or by her own workout needs? A relationship as intimate as that of personal trainer and client mandates good camaraderie, and can even evolve into a comfortable friendship, but it must keep your fitness interests foremost, in first place. "He or she should act like a professional," says Pam Germain. "You wouldn't want to go to a psychologist and have them tell you their problems, and you don't want a personal trainer who's just concerned about his own fitness."

A good trainer is interested in helping you maintain a balanced, healthy lifestyle in addition to exercise. He or she will keep a record of your workouts and update your medical history periodically; put workout methods in writing and explain the reasoning behind them; encourage you to ask questions and take notes on anything you don't understand. And get along well with you.

WHAT MATTERS, WHAT DOESN'T

What Matters

• A gym that's easy to get to.

• A trainer who's appropriately certified.

• Proper footwear.

• A variety of resources to let your fitness program "grow."

What Doesn't

• Expensive, long-term training contracts.

• Technical expertise that isn't personalized to your needs.

• Matching the pace of other exercisers in a class.

• "Today only" gym membership offers—don't be pressured into a choice.

How Much, How Often

Your first session with a trainer is likely to be more talk than action, including the health screening and other evaluation you need before launching into the exercise. After that, the frequency with which you'll be meeting is entirely up to you and your pocketbook. For some, the more, the better, and the personal trainer can become a daily workout buddy to spur you on.

At the minimum, two to three sessions over a one- to three-week period are usually enough to get a good grasp of what you're doing. Schedule a follow-up a few weeks later to check your progress and update your routine.

The rate you'll be charged depends on the length of the workout, the trainer's experience, and where you'll be training—not only because fees vary greatly throughout the country, but a trainer working out of a club, or on its staff, will have a different fee structure than one working on his or her own.

A survey of IDEA personal trainer members revealed full-fee sessions costing anywhere from under $25 to over $70, with an average of $41. Good news: Only 62 percent of their clients paid the full fee. A preset package of sessions, group workouts, and other incentives can bring the price down. (As with gyms, most people sign up in January, fresh from their New Year's resolutions, so you might get a better deal during slower summer months.) Ask about cancellation policies when you negotiate your agreement. Some will charge for missed appointments if a certain amount of advance notice has not been given.

"A good trainer will help a person find an activity that they really, really enjoy," says NAFC's

Germain. "People think, 'What's better, lifting weights or jogging?' There's really nothing good or bad, it's what you will enjoy and keep doing.

"We already have enough punishment in our lives. So if you're working on your body, why not make it one of the pleasant parts?"

Classes

From meditation to military-type training, health club exercise classes offer the motivational and leadership advantages of a personal trainer at considerably lower cost. Group energy and team spirit don't hurt, either.

Many of the activities discussed in chapter 3 are available in classrooom settings: aquatics, slide- and step-training, workouts with exercise bands or stability balls. An IDEA survey found increases in lifestyle-betterment programs in how to stop smoking or lose weight, as well as fitness programs like ballroom dance and ballet, walking, circuit training, tai chi, martial arts, and one of the most popular, yoga. "Yoga is part of the whole mind-body movement that is very popular today," says Cathy Masterson McNeil, of International Health, Racquet and Sportsclub Association.

On the other end of the intensity spectrum is the boot camp approach to training, the "tough love" of the exercise world, where a leader drills participants, pushing them to the max. "The people who like this are the people who are very athletic," says McNeil. "Or

Top Five Club Users

Here's who's visiting health clubs (in number of average visits per year):

Men, age 65+	139
Men, age 45–54	114
Women, age 65+	108
Men, age 25–34	95
Men, age 55–64	91

Source: International Health, Racquet and Sportsclub Association (data for 1996)

Gyms and health clubs aren't for everyone. But for those who thrive on energetic surroundings at a dedicated exercise locale, they can provide levels of training, equipment, and activity that can be a challenge to reach on your own. Professional trainers provide another option—at a fitness center or in individual sessions tailored to your needs. Exercise classes are a middle-ground alternative, offering some of the benefits of both trainers and the gym. Whether you choose one, or either of the others, or a combination of the three, there's a wide range of fitness options to better your program and your chances of success.

people who think, 'I need someone to kick me in the pants.'"

Other forms of equipment-based group exercise, like indoor cycling, are spreading rapidly at fitness centers as well, from treading (treadmills), to crewing (rowing machines), to power pumping (free weights).

Some gyms include the price of certain classes in the membership dues; others levy a tuition per session or course. But you don't necessarily have to be a gym member to participate in these activities, which are also often available at local recreation centers, through adult education programs, or as individual offerings at a health club.

Look for a teacher as you would a personal trainer, being sure they're skilled not just in the exercise itself but in teaching it as well.

CHAPTER 5

....

Working Out On Your Own

While many people prefer to pump their iron and their cardiovascular systems at fitness centers, others opt for a more secluded, or scenic, workout locale. If the sound of a roomful of machines whirring and the sight of a crowd of exercisers perspiring brings the phrase "sweat shop" to mind; if you don't want someone else selecting your workout music; or if you just don't want to be surrounded by other people before you get that body toned and shaped, there are many other alternatives to fit you.

The Pros and Cons

Working out on your own—at home, around it, or in the general neighborhood—can be more convenient, less expensive, and, for many, a more pleasant experience than going to a gym. And the more pleasant the exercise, the more likely you are to keep it up.

You can convert the time you'd spend in transit into valuable workout time, use a fraction of the money you'd spend on gym membership in exchange for some sessions with a personal trainer, and never have to wait in line for a piece of equipment again. Another valuable benefit: If you can enlist family members to join you—or if they've enlisted *you*—the whole household can become healthier and happier; plus, if you're surrounded by round-the-clock support like that, it's easier for everyone in the family to live the fitness lifestyle.

On the downside: The cost and space required

for the range of equipment available at a fitness center puts it out of the question for most, and developing a well-balanced program on your own requires guidance and ingenuity. Inclement weather can put a crimp in an outdoor walking routine, as can a lack of sidewalks, or safe neighborhoods through which to walk. Without supervision, you run greater risks of harm. And if you live in an apartment, the downstairs neighbor might object to some of the more energetic aspects of your aerobic routine.

Lastly, but hardly least, there's the distraction factor: Not all families *are* supportive, and some may even try to sabotage your efforts to assuage their own guilt over not exercising. Will you be able to focus on fitness when your best friend—or the TV in the corner—calls? Without a personal trainer or fitness class instructor, you're not only lacking crucial professional guidance but the motivating influence he or she can provide.

Before you decide working out on your own is for you, be sure you have:

• The self-discipline to do it;

• The space to do it in;

• A solid understanding of a well-rounded fitness program, including backup plans when bad weather strikes;

• Supportive family members—or adequate time away from less supportive types.

F.Y.I.

Americans use a variety of fitness equipment at home (in percentage of those who own home equipment):

Free weights 35.6

Treadmills 25.0

Stationary cycles 22.5

Spot toners 12.3

Cross-country ski machines 8.1

Stair-climbing machines 6.7

Multi-station home gyms 5.6

Aerobic riders 5.6

Cardiovascular gliding machines . . 3.8

Rowing machines . 3.0

Walkers 2.2

Other 3.5

Source: Fitness Products Council

Watch Out While You Work Out

Working out on your own puts the burden of safety precautions squarely on your own deltoids. While everyone should exercise caution with every exercise, going it alone calls for an extra measure of care.

And that doesn't just apply to heavy apparatus that can fall on your head. Overexertion of your heart can be dangerous, as can, alas, a run around the block.

"We tell people we're going out into the desert for a hike," says J. David Bergeron, Ph.D., a former emergency medical technician who's an instructional technologist, and author of *The Coaches' Guide to Sport Injuries* (Human Kinetics), among others. "Let them know you're going for a jog and will be back at a certain time."

Better yet, especially if you're planning a strenuous workout, enlist a friend or family member to join you, and you'll not only be safer but more motivated. (The number-one reason most people stop working out on their home fitness equipment: They don't like working out alone.) If no one's available, keep a phone on hand—indoors or out—in case you fall and can't get up.

Selecting a dedicated exercise area in which to work out will help keep you focused on what you're doing there. Don't banish yourself to a mildewy basement or anywhere else you don't like to be. Choose a place that's roomy and pleasant, with good lighting and ventilation.

Go for safety: If you're exercising on a carpeted area, be sure it doesn't have folds on which you can trip, or loops or fringes on which you can catch. On the floor? Watch that perspiration doesn't leave it wet and slippery. Special aerobics boards made of springy wood are good for absorbing impact, and exercise mats can cushion your back. Also, be sure no obstacles—tables, hanging light fixtures, or that precious Ming vase—will get in your way.

And remember that you're not the only one who can be hurt. While you're concentrating on your own fitness, be sure to keep an eye out for what your children or pets—or the neighbors' children or pets—are doing as well.

"The greater the concentration on yourself," says Bergeron, "the less the concentration on overseeing anyone or anything else."

Working Out Outdoors

Taking to the outdoors can be more scenic and interesting than working out within your own four walls. But then you have to deal with the elements: In the rain, for instance, visibility and traction are impaired; running fifteen minutes on a hot day can raise your body temperature as much as five degrees above normal; working out in the cold, when muscles are tighter and stiffer, puts them at greater risk of tear. Here are some other things to keep in mind.

In the Heat

When the temperature is up, take the level and length of your workout down. As body temperature rises, the risk of heat stroke and heat exhaus-

SMART MONEY

"Always have fun," says strength trainer John Abdo. "My slogan is 'My body is my hobby.' Like most other hobbies, you involve yourself with it. Take a class, rent movies, go to the library. *Learning* yourself saves a lot of frustration, time, and energy, and it boosts your confidence and encourages you when you see results."

F.Y.I.

Sun protection factor (SPF) of the average T-shirt: 6–9

SPF of the same T-shirt wet, from swimming or profuse sweat 3

Source: The New York Times

tion do, too. The heart beats faster, muscles fatigue more quickly, and performance declines.

• **Be aware of the humidity level.** While a ninety-degree temperature is relatively safe at 10 percent humidity, the heat stress with 50 percent humidity would be the same as if it were ninety-six degrees. In the summer, or in tropical climates, exercising in the early morning or evening hours is best.

• **Dress cool.** Loose-fitting, lightweight, light-colored clothing—the less of it, the better—allows heat to dissipate from your skin. Avoiding cotton and other water-absorbing fabrics will keep you cooler and more comfortable; special lines of clothing such as Solumbra from Sun Precautions, Inc., have built-in protection from cancer-causing ultraviolet (UV) rays.

• **Use sunscreen.** Everywhere. Because the kind of clothing that keeps you cool can also allow UV rays to reach the skin, sunscreen needs to be applied all over, not just on exposed skin. Choose a sun protection factor (SPF) no lower than 15, and higher if you burn easily or will be outside for extended periods of time. Certain antibiotics can increase sensitivity to the sun as well; read labels and heed warnings.

• **Wear sunglasses and a hat.** Your eyes and head are not exempt from UV damage. Opt for shades that block 90 to 100 percent of UV rays, cover the whole eye, and won't jiggle around with activity. A brimmed hat or cap can protect your neck and face as well as the top of your head.

• **Drink lots of water.** Before, during, and after

exercise. The hotter it is, the more you'll sweat, and the greater the likelihood of dehydration, which leaves your body's cooling systems impaired. Don't wait until you're thirsty, either—your body won't signal dehydration until you're well on the way. Six to eight ounces of fluid is recommended every fifteen to twenty minutes you exercise. A good guide: Weigh yourself before and after exercising (preferably not in sweat-soaked clothes), then drink two cups of water for each pound lost. (More about water in chapter 6.)

In the Cold

Wind chill is to the cold as humidity is to the heat, heightening the effect of the numbers on the thermometer. When the body loses more heat than it produces, you risk frostbite (see below) and hypothermia, which in severe cases can cause rigid muscles, dark and puffy skin, irregular heart-beat and breathing, and unconsciousness. Listen to the *whole* weather report.

• **Dress warm.** Layers of loose-fitting clothing can keep warm air in and allow sweat to pass through. Again, avoid heavy cotton or tightly woven material, which absorb water and don't allow a layer of dry air near the skin. Instead, you might opt for new sports-wear fabrics, which have the layers built in. Scarves or masks can warm the air you're inhaling, but if it's that cold, it might be wiser to stay inside.

• **Keep your extremities cozy.** Head, neck, hands, and feet are especially susceptible to harm when temperatures plummet and blood is drawn away from them to keep the center of the body warm.

SMART SOURCES

Bicycle Helmet Safety
 Institute
4611 Seventh St. S.
Arlington, VA 22204
703-486-0100
www.bhsi.org.

According to the Bicycle Helmet Safety Institute (BHSI), the helmet advocacy program of the Washington Area Bicyclist Association, head injury causes 75 percent of the 900 annual deaths from bicycle crashes. Helmets could prevent 88 percent of those injuries.

 BHSI volunteers provide helmet information and work on national helmet-standard committees.

With up to 50 percent of the body's heat loss coming from the head, a hat is a must. Gloves can help prevent tissue damage to the hands and fingers, but to protect your feet you have to keep the rest of your body warm.

• **Watch for frostbite.** The severity of frostbite is hard to gauge until hours after thawing. Gray or yellowish patches; waxy, pale areas that turn red or purple; or blisters are signs that you need medical attention. Until then, get to a warm place, remove any constrictive clothing, and, if the frostbitten area is partially thawed, place it in warm water (102 to 106 degrees) for twenty to forty minutes. *Do not:* Use water hotter than 106 degrees or cooler than 100 degrees; rub or massage the area; or rub it with ice or snow.

At Night

It's sad but true that anyone out at night for any reason runs safety risks. For exercisers, there's more than the chance of violence, there's the collision factor: You can't see who's coming, and they can't see you.

Avoid dark, narrow roadways, and wear reflective clothing—a vest, or arm and leg bands—or reflective tape to increase visibility. On bikes, front and rear lights and reflectors are more than a good idea: The Consumer Product Safety Commission requires reflectors on all new models—in front and rear, on pedals, and on side rims or wheels. Many states require front and rear lights. Small battery-operated lamps strapped to your legs will also help. And, day or night, *never* forget your helmet.

City Streets, Country Roads

Reduce the risks of falls, sprains, and other accidents by keeping to smooth, paved, away-from-traffic surfaces. The best running surface is a cinder track or soft-surface running path, but asphalt is better than grass, which usually has more gullies, rocks, and other hazards. Shun streets, driveways, or areas covered by water, sand, gravel, or dirt.

In urban areas, runners should stay as far as possible from car exhaust fumes, and keep the headset volume down to hear honking horns. And if you opt to go off the beaten path into that gorgeous country setting, remember, there may be a reason why that road is less traveled. Don't go into uncharted territory, and wear plenty of insecticide.

Making the Investment

Americans spent $4.8 billion for home exercise equipment in 1996, according to the Fitness Products Council (FPC). And 35 percent of those who owned equipment aren't using it anymore. The moral of the story: No dumbbell, no treadmill, no multi-station gym is worth the paper on which its receipt is printed if it's not right for you.

"Play It Again Sports has built an industry around Americans' love of buying equipment and not using it," says Lynn Allen, the FPC spokesperson and certified trainer who helped President and Mrs. Clinton redo the White House fitness room. "The single biggest mistake is to assume

F.Y.I.

Here's what Americans spend on fitness equipment (in millions of dollars*):

Treadmills.... $1,450

Aerobic riders... $800

Cross-country ski machines ... $510

Abdominal exercisers..... $450

Multi-station home gyms.... $410

Stationary cycles........ $340

Stair-climbing machines...... $260

Free weights ... $250

Benches $214

Other ** $200

* Estimated from wholesale figures

** Hand weights, jump ropes, rowing machines, and other devices

Source: Fitness Products Council

that *buying* equipment will guarantee that it's going to be used."

The most important piece of equipment: an education.

"Have a plan in place," says Allen, who provided the same advice to the Clintons, who went with a good mix of aerobic and resistance-training machines. (Hillary likes the recumbent cycle; Bill balances his jogging routine with upper-body strength workouts.) "Don't just see a late-night infomercial and decide that [what it's advertising is] for you."

Will machinery be supplementing an outdoor fitness or class program, or provide your entire workout? Will you be working alone, or with a trainer who can guide you through a more complex routine?

The kind of home gym you have also depends on where you are on the fitness scale. If you're currently leading a sedentary life, any step is an important one, and you can easily make improvements just by running up and down the stairs more often, or doing garden work, or stretches, or jumping jacks if you don't have neighbors downstairs. If you have any physical limitations, check with your physician.

"Once you identify what you want—establish a short-term goal—you can identify the kind of map that will get you there," says John Abdo, strength and conditioning specialist, author of *Body Engineering*, and an Olympic strength trainer who helped lead speed skater Bonnie Blair to those gold medal wins. "Once you get there, it turns into a lifestyle."

Books, magazines, videos, television shows, and an ocean of surfable web sites provide a deluge of information on general fitness and realistic goal-setting. Then, when you know what you want and are willing to give what it takes to get it, you can set up a program—and the pieces of equipment—that are right for you.

How to Buy Exercise Equipment

Most health clubs—even if you don't belong—will gladly give you a tour of the facility and all its machinery, if not a full day's trial run. A good first step is to consult a professional trainer, who can help you determine a good, sound plan. Often, he or she will be able to make recommendations, not only of what sort of equipment, but of the model and style that's right for you. (Find out whether the trainer has any commercial interest in a store or manufacturer before blindly following advice.) Following are some helpful basic buying tips.

• **Penny wise, pound foolish.** Don't skimp on a quality piece of equipment for a roomful of shoddy machinery. When you're making an investment in yourself, durability, safety, and the features that will keep you using what you buy are invaluable.

• **Try before you buy.** Test-drive a wide range of equipment, with an array of features, to see what you enjoy most. If you know someone with home gym equipment, ask to try it out, or visit a gym on a friend's guest privileges to see what different

If Cost Is the Object

Gym equipment can be pricey. Common household items or daily activities can fill in for some.

Instead of	Use
Dumbbells	Soup cans, books, paperweights
Stationary cycle	Your bicycle
Treadmill	The sidewalk
Step machines	Your staircase
Exercise mat	Pile of quilts

SMART SOURCES

ConsumerMatters
5820 Oberlin Dr.
Suite 102
San Diego, CA 92121
800-529-8227
www.acefitness.org

This publication of the American Council on Exercise (ACE) offers a series of articles on specific types of exercise equipment based on ACE consumer evaluation and health and fitness product research.

Sporting Goods Manu-
  facturers Association
200 Castlewood Dr.
North Palm Beach, FL
  33408
561-842-4100
www.sportlink.com

This nonprofit trade association that begat the Fitness Products Council has a web site that provides a behind-the-scenes look at the exercise and sports equipment industry, including new-product updates and referrals to manufacturers.

pieces are like. Then, when you're ready to make a purchase, show up in exercise clothes and workout shoes, prepared for a mini-workout on different models of the machine. Keep in mind the equipment's ease of use, smoothness or vibration, and even styling you prefer.

• **Consider your space.** "Some people want something they can slide under a bed," says Lynn Allen. But remember, number one: If you can move a piece of equipment around that easily, it's not very sturdy. And number two: Out of sight, out of mind. If it slides under the bed, says Allen, "it'll stay under that bed." Be sure to take measurements of the space you will use (including the doorways through which the equipment needs to pass), and take workout-room TVs or stereos into account.

• **Buy from a specialty retail store.** A reputable retailer that specializes in exercise equipment will more than make up for the difference in price you'll find at the local discount mega-retailer. Not only will you find greater selection and have the chance to try out the machines, but the experience of trained salespeople can be invaluable. Ask lots of questions about features, models, and manufacturers, and check the store's installation, maintenance, and service plans.

• **Keep others in mind.** If other people in your household will be using the equipment, be sure it will accommodate their weight, height, and fitness needs. The more of a workout the workout equipment will get, the more sturdy it needs to be.

• **Listen.** Especially if you're buying a used item, listen to hear that it's running smoothly and not squeaking. Is it too loud to hear your stereo or TV while you use it? Or will it bother others in the house? Or next door?

• **Check the manufacturer.** Make sure that the product has a good warranty (generally, the longer the warranty, the better the quality) and that there is a readily available customer service line to answer any questions you may have.

The Wrong Stuff: Let the Buyer Beware

In its brochure "Fraudulent Health Claims: Don't Be Fooled," the Federal Trade Commission teams with the U.S. Food and Drug Administration to warn us of unproven, fraudulently marketed, and sometimes useless health-care products and treatments on the market today. Applicable to exercise equipment as well as miracle diet cures, it's good advice that can not only save us a lot of money but, more important, protect us against serious harm. Watch for claims that:

• Sound too good to be true—they probably are.

• Promise quick and effective cure-alls for a wide range of ailments or for undiagnosed pain.

• Include phrases like *scientific breakthrough, miraculous cure, secret ingredient,* or *ancient remedy.*

• Say the medical profession or research scientists have conspired to suppress the product.

• Boast undocumented case histories claiming amazing results.

• Involve products available from only one source, and require payment in advance.

Finally, don't rely on promises of a "money-back guarantee." Many fly-by-night operators will not be around to respond to a refund request.

SMART DEFINITIONS

Walking/running shoes
Flex at the ball of the foot, support the heel, and provide traction to move you along. Off-trail walkers need extra stability; power and fitness walkers require extra cushioning.

Aerobics shoes
Crucial cushioning and shock absorption, good arch and side support, and sufficiently thick upper leather or strap support to provide forefoot stability and prevent slips.

Basketball shoes
Lots of ankle support and shock absorption.

• **Open with care.** Save packaging material in case the product needs to be returned for servicing, or moving plans appear down the road.

What to Buy

As we said before, there's no need to make a major investment at the start—exercise mats, a sturdy weight bench, a set of light dumbbells, and appropriate footwear provide a sufficient foundation. Unless you're the type whose feet need to follow your wallet (studies have found that the more expensive the equipment, the longer it's used), overspending can exhaust you both financially and mentally, and you run the risk of having a very expensive piece of garage furniture.

If you decide to go ahead with major purchases, be sure to check that electrical outlets are conveniently located and can accommodate the equipment (customized wiring can cost). An extra-thick carpet pad and tightly woven short pile indoor/outdoor carpeting provide a good base to work on; tweedlike combinations can hide oils from machinery, or dirt and rubber from shoes. When buying cardiovascular equipment, watch for electronic conveniences packed into lower-end machines at the expense of overall durability, and buy rubber mats specifically designed to fit under each piece. Resistance equipment should have sound construction and versatile settings for a range of exercise.

Best Bets for Cardiovascular Fitness

Treadmill. The top-ranked home aerobic equipment for years running is available with a wide array of features, from varying incline to feedback on time, distance, and calories burned. Look for a wide, long, stable belt that can accommodate your stride and weight; emergency shutoff; and slow-start speeds; as well as quality in the drive train, belt, and deck. Cushioning features can help lessen the impact on feet and knees.

Stationary cycle. With a small learning curve, stationary cycles are easy to use, and low impact. Available in upright or recumbent styles, some cycles come with movable handles to work your upper body as you go, and you should make sure the one you buy has a comfortable, adjustable seat, interchangeable seat posts, and adjustable handles and toe straps. Less costly "trainers" allow you to convert your outdoor bicycle for indoor use.

Step machines. Whether stair-climbing or pedal-pushed, these can provide a good workout, though with a larger learning curve than treadmills and cycles. Machines with independent steps require more coordination. Look for steps parallel to the floor at all times, and a stable railing to grasp.

Elliptical trainers. *The* hot new category of machines—a cross between stair-climbing, cross-country skiing, and jogging—which FPC's Lynn Allen calls "fabulous" for the machines' short learning curve, extremely low impact, and cardio-vascular effectiveness. "Some clubs have a thirty-minute limit on it and people wait their turn like vultures," she says. "You know it's popular." Look for changeable elevation; feedback; smooth, elliptical motion; and a big, nonslip footbed. Some models provide upper-body workouts, as well.

SMART DEFINITIONS

Cycling shoes
Provide support across the arch and instep. Cross-training or combination cycling-hiking shoes work for the average rider; specific racing and mountain-biking shoes are for serious enthusiasts.

Tennis and racquet sports shoes
For side-to-side motion, twisting, pivoting, and quick stopping and starting that stress foot and ankle, these shoes need appropriate "give," and well-padded heels and toes.

Resistance-Training Equipment

Free weights. A set of light dumbbells will allow a good range of resistance for upper-body exercise. Available in weights as low as one pound, and at low cost, a good beginner's set might consist of three-, five-, and eight-pound weights (different exercises present different levels of challenge). When you can do ten to twelve repetitions easily, move on to heavier resistance. A vertical dumbbell rack provides space-efficient storage.

Benches. A sturdy, high-quality weight bench that adjusts to incline through several positions, ending in an upright position, can allow greater range of motion during weight-training exercise. Be sure to check width, length, and cushioning for comfort.

Ankle and sandbag weights. Not to be worn while walking or running, ankle weights add resistance and challenge for lower-body workouts, while sandbag weights offer a comfortable way to increase the intensity of leg-lifts and other exercises. And both kinds of weights are inexpensive.

Multi-station gyms. Multi-station home gyms allow safe and effective exercise of every major muscle group, and can be as compact as four feet by eight feet by four feet. The type recommended by the American Council on Exercise

Signs That You Should See a Doctor

• A change in the way you stand or walk.

• Pain or swelling lasting more than three days.

• Any kind of internal bleeding.

• Unusual, increasing, or sharp pain.

• Vomiting, or pain after eating.

• Fever.

• Infection.

• Warning signals of a heart attack: Uncomfortable pressure, fullness, or pain in the center of the chest lasting more than a few minutes; pain spreading to the shoulders, neck, or arms; chest discomfort with lightheadedness, fainting, sweating, nausea, or shortness of breath. (And men aren't the only ones affected—heart attacks are the number-one killer of women.)

(ACE) are machines with adjustable weight stacks that use cables and pulleys. The ACE warns against rubberized resistance machines, whose resistance is not always uniform, and which can break down. A major advantage of weight-stack gyms: They are generally more adjustable to accommodate a variety of user sizes, and are safer to use without a spotter.

"Multi-gym means multi-purpose, and with some, portable or fixed attachments allow you to do twenty different exercises," says John Abdo. Although they provide a more-than-adequate home workout, they are inferior to single-station units at a health club. Says Abdo, "The one-man band never sounds as good as a full orchestra."

Flexibility-Training Equipment

Many books and videos can help you develop a flexibility program based on body weight and a few household props (such as door frames or sturdy railings). A full-length mirror can help you watch for proper form. A few major companies make flexibility devices, but in ACE's opinion, most don't address this category adequately.

On-Screen Education

People working out on their own are in particular need of good sources of advice, many of which are as close as their own television or computer screen.

Exercise Videos

Every celebrity seems to have one, and others have become celebrities *from* having one.

"Anyone who talks biceps and triceps, and anaerobic and aerobic, can look like an expert," says John Abdo. Having a vocabulary is not the same as having knowledge, though, and moreover, jargon-laden instruction can interfere with the ability to teach.

Jane Fonda and Cindy Crawford aside, look for videos led by certified fitness professionals who include timeouts for heart-rate checking and rest, and stress a balanced program of fitness over the "all you need is weight loss and life will be wonderful" approach. Just as no one piece of equipment can meet all your fitness needs, neither can one video. Your best bet: three good basic workouts—one aerobic, one resistance, and one featuring flexibility routines. In each area, select a level of training that suits you.

Abdo, whose weekly *TN 2000* television show broadcasts training and nutrition advice nationwide, warns viewers of all shows, videos, and, for that matter, exercise class instructors to proceed with caution:

"If someone's doing something fast and explosive, do it slow and controlled so your body can become accustomed to the movement first. Never compete with the other guy or gal who's jumping or bounding around and who's been doing this for years."

With videos, remember the pause button, and use it. Or follow along at a slower pace.

At the Computer

If your computer skills are in good shape, you might want to try health and fitness software and CD-ROMs, which are inexpensive and offer customizable workouts, track your progress, and even bring "virtual trainers" right to your computer screen. Some programs come complete with skinfold calipers and tape measures; one even includes a packet of whey protein and a motivation tape.

The range of features varies by product, and can include text, audio, and video information, as well as databases in the areas of nutrition and mental health. Some record entries for single or multiple users; others allow Internet interface.

For those with strong cyber muscles, surfing the Web can provide a workout in and of itself. Just plug a key word—or up to five words—into your search engine of choice, and you're off.

Remember, though, that anyone can put anything they want on the Web, so stick with reputable, established sites. A good general guide: Sites ending in ".edu" are usually universities; ".gov" indicates government sites; and ".org" denotes nonprofit organizations. And watch for blatant commercialism wherever you are.

Megasites such as the Internet Fitness Resource (rampages.onramp.net/~chaz) and Good Health Web (www.social.com/health/nhic/data) can refer you to literally thousands of health and fitness sources in the area of your choice. Is your trainer certified by the American College of Sports Medicine? Check out that site (www.acsm.org) to learn what's involved. Magazines such as *The Physician and Sportsmedicine* (www.physsportsmed.com) are available on-line. In addition, there are sites dedicated to specific fitness activities (the Road Run-

SMART MONEY

Sprains, blisters, and shin splints are among the injuries traceable to inappropriate, or improperly fitted athletic shoes. "The design of the shoe should be geared toward the sport," says Perry H. Julien, D.P.M., of the American Academy of Podiatric Sports Medicine. "With running and walking you're going straight ahead; with tennis, side-to-side." Shoes should be appropriate for the activity. Julien recommends you:

• Shop at an athletic shoe store in the afternoon, when feet are slightly swelled; wear the same socks and foot-support devices you'd wear during your workout.

• Bring your old shoes so the fitter can read the wear patterns.

• Replace shoes every 300 to 600 miles.

ners Club of America, at www.rrca.org) as well as sites with a number of links to a wide variety of special-interest groups (Woman's Sports Page, at fiat.gslis.utexas.edu/~lewisa/womsprt.html).

Some web sites allow you to download information for free that you'd have to pay for if requested by mail; others grant access to material otherwise available only to members.

Remember, some computer software and web sites come from people with more computer expertise than health and fitness knowledge, and some fitness professionals lack computer finesse. As always, take the source of the advice into account.

Common Exercise Injuries and How to Treat Them

You'll hear it again and again and again: Exercising without proper warm-up, cool-down, and stretching; overdoing it; using improper form; and not wearing the proper footwear can get you hurt.

For most injuries—from runner's knee to tennis elbow—follow three basic tips: (1) Stop what you're doing and don't start again until you're feeling better; (2) take over-the-counter anti-inflammatory medications such as aspirin or ibuprofen if you need something to relieve the pain; and (3) to reduce swelling and speed recovery, "RICE":

• **Rest.** Give the injured body part some time off.

• **Ice.** Apply cold compresses for periods of up to

twenty minutes but not more than twice in an hour.

• **Compression.** Use an elastic bandage (always wrap from far to near), making sure the wrap isn't too tight.

• **Elevation.** Raise the injured part of the body to minimize swelling and help circulation.

Remember, self-diagnosis can be faulty, so if the problem doesn't get better, or worsens, seek professional care.

Achilles Tendon and Calf Pain

The tendon attached to the back of the heel bone and the large muscles in the back of the legs can cause feelings of pain and tightness when inflamed. Stretching the calf muscles gently and gradually before and after your workout can help.

Athlete's Foot

The burning, itching, scaling inflammation and blisters that commonly start between the toes are caused by a fungus that is usually contracted in showers, locker rooms, and pools, and thrives in dark, moist places, like inside your shoe. And it's not limited to the foot: Touching an infected area can transmit the infection to other parts of the body as well. Keep feet clean and dry by dusting foot powder in shoes and socks, avoid walking barefoot, and try an over-the-counter remedy. Advanced cases may require a prescription cure.

Motivation Strategies for Those Who Work Out Alone

• Get a friend to join you.

• Set—and keep to—a schedule.

• Have a just-for-workout set of clothing.

• Do your exercise routine in a dedicated place.

• Keep distractions away—by working out when there are less of them or in a place where they can't find you. Turn off the phone.

Forget the Gimmicks

Some of the most popular miracle devices on the market today promise to rid your body of the flab around the stomach, or "abs." First, remember: No localized exercise will get rid of excess fat—only cardiovascular exercise burns fat, and it does that in places determined by your genes, not your activity. But to strengthen and tone your midsection, you don't need those gimmicks; just crunches.

• **For a basic crunch:** Lie on the floor with knees bent and arms across your chest. Keeping your back flat on the floor, lift your shoulders and chest several inches as you exhale, then inhale as you slowly release.

• **To work obliques (the side-of-the-stomach muscles):** Lift one shoulder (not elbow) toward the opposite knee as you exhale, then inhale as you slowly release. Repeat on the other side.

• **To work lower abs:** Bring knees up toward the chest, forming a right angle with the body. Using only the lower abs (not legs or hips), bring knees slightly toward your chest as you exhale, then inhale as you slowly release. Note: This is a small movement; don't try to bring your knees up to your face.

Start with ten repetitions of each exercise, and as your muscles get stronger, increase the number, or try doing it with your arms extended behind your head. And *always* use proper technique: *Don't* pull on your neck; keep the chin a fist's distance from the chest. *Don't* use jerking motions; stay slow and controlled.

Back and Muscle Pain

Pain in the middle or lower portion of the back usually indicates a strained muscle. The RICE approach, moderate bed rest (sometimes it feels better to gently stretch your muscles), and pain relievers are the best treatment.

Blisters

These friction problems present an age-old question: To pop or not to pop? Although theories vary, in general: If the blister isn't large, don't. Apply an antiseptic, cover with a moleskin or adhesive bandage, and let it take care of itself. Burst a large blister with a sterile needle and a few punctures to its "roof"; drain the fluid as thoroughly as possible before soaking it in warm water, applying an antiseptic, and bandaging. Never remove the roof.

Shin Splints

These injuries to the front and inside of the leg are probably the most common exercise-induced lower-body injury, as it's the muscles attached to the shin bone that move the foot up and down. Although the term is used inaccurately to describe many kinds of injury, "tibial stress syndrome" or "tibial fasciitis" is usually caused by running on hard surfaces, overstriding, or muscle imbalance. RICE, reduce stride length, and reduce your exercise time and intensity by half until the pain subsides.

Strains and Sprains

Strains happen when you overstretch or tear tendons, the part of the muscle that attaches to the bone. Sprains involve torn or overstretched ligaments, the tissue that joins bones together. Immediate treatment with the RICE technique to reduce swelling helps.

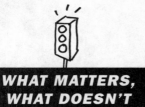

WHAT MATTERS, WHAT DOESN'T

What Matters

- Safety.
- A dedicated exercise area.
- Setting and following a workout schedule.
- Self-discipline.
- Quality, appropriate equipment.

What Doesn't

- Keeping up with the person on the video.
- Having a roomful of equipment.
- Sophisticated web sites sponsored by an unreliable source.

Stress Fractures

Unlike *fractures,* which require immediate medical care, *stress fractures* are incomplete cracks in the bone caused by overuse, and call for complete rest. Women are more likely to develop stress fractures than men.

Tennis Elbow

Not just for tennis players, this inflammation of the muscles in the tendon and forearm that attach to the elbow also occurs in golfers, lifters, rowers, and others who use strenuous or repetitive movement of the forearm. Exercises and stretches to increase forearm strength and flexibility appear to be the best overall treatment, and for tennis players, a different size or type of racquet or grip can help. Tennis elbow straps can decrease stress on the injured elbow, but if the problem isn't really tennis elbow, a strap can keep it from healing by allowing continued, uncorrected play.

THE BOTTOM LINE

The right place to work out can mean the difference between a successful fitness program and one that never quite manages to get anywhere. For many, with its convenience, privacy, and lower cost, there's no place like home. Not only is it where your heart (and muscle tone) is, but your efforts can prompt your whole household to better health. With a session or two with a certified personal trainer, and the right equipment, you can have the best of both fitness worlds. The keys are self-motivation, self-discipline, and familiarity with proper equipment, safety, and technique.

Food for Fitness

A good exercise program needs food to fuel it. A balanced eating plan that supplies the right amount of nutrients and energy is essential for achieving and maintaining strength, flexibility, and endurance. In addition to meeting their basic needs as human beings, physically active people have to be especially sure they take in enough fluids and low-fat, high-carbohydrate foods to replenish the fluids and energy they use. And, as with physical activity, even minor changes in how you do that can make a difference.

An Active Lifestyle's Special Needs

What you eat and the way you eat can greatly affect your body-fat level as well as your overall health and well-being. And that will affect how well your exercise program succeeds.

Although a very different set of needs really only comes into play at the high end of the exercise scale—for marathoners and competitive athletes—people exercising for fitness still need to take special care to meet their basic needs: their bread and water, almost literally.

"I always try to encourage people to be aware of fluid consumption and make more effort to increase carbohydrate intake, the energy source that muscles favor," says Chris Rosenbloom, Ph.D., R.D., associate professor of nutrition at Georgia State University and director of sports nutrition for the Georgia Tech Athletic Association.

When you eat in relation to when you exercise

matters as well. By "fueling up" with a multinutrient meal a few hours before a workout, you give your body enough time for the food to be processed, and you won't be focusing on your hunger instead of your workout. "If you're doing an early-morning activity and don't have that time span, try a carbohydrate-based, light meal," says Leslie Bonci, R.D., of the American Dietetic Association (ADA), at Allegheny General Hospital in Pittsburgh. "A piece of toast or a handful of dried cereal will give a little carbohydrate to work on but not enough to cause tremendous discomfort while you're working out."

If you're exerting yourself for more than an hour at a time, follow up with some carbohydrates and protein shortly afterward to replenish the body's stores.

What Is Metabolism? And What Do Calories Have to Do with It?

Every minute we live and breathe, chemical reactions are going on in every cell of the body. Some of them use energy, others release it. The rate at which the body uses energy is what we mean when we talk about metabolism. That energy is measured in what scientists call kilocalories, and what we call calories. In other words, calories are not evil little things contained in the foods we eat, but good measures of how much energy it takes to process the food.

The minimum amount of energy (or calories) you need to keep functioning when you're awake

SMART SOURCES

American Dietetic
  Association
216 W. Jackson Blvd.
Suite 800
Chicago, IL 60606
800-366-1655
900-225-5267
www.eatright.org

The nation's largest organization of food and nutrition professionals offers easily accessible, objective food and nutrition information. Check the web site, or call the Consumer Nutrition Hotline at 800-366-1655 for messages and fact sheets, or for a referral to a registered dietitian near you. For customized answers by a registered dietitian, call 900-CALL-AN-RD ($1.95 for the first minute, 95 cents per minute after that).

is your basal metabolic rate, which is just slightly lower than your resting metabolic rate, the rate under quiet resting conditions. In other words, we're always burning calories—whether we're just breathing, digesting food, or crossing the finish line of a race. The resting metabolic rate alone can account for up to 60 to 75 percent of the total daily energy we use.

To find out your metabolic rate directly, you would need to use a human calorimeter, a large, airtight, thermally insulated chamber that allows your heat energy production to be calculated over time. Simpler methods are based on oxygen consumption, or estimates from formulas that consider your weight, height, sex, and age. (These are the sort of estimates that go into those tables that tell us how many calories we burn on average while performing an activity.) An average man weighing 150 pounds, for example, will use approximately 65 calories per hour while sleeping, 350 while walking, and 900 while running. A 120-pound woman will burn 60 calories while sitting quietly, 350 while cycling, and 550 while swimming. The calories we don't use up are stored as body fat, with 3,500 calories adding up to one pound of fat.

How many calories our body needs to support itself depends on how our metabolism runs. Bodies with higher metabolisms require more calories to keep going (these belong to the often-envied types of people who can't seem to eat enough to keep up); others seem to subsist on a minimum of calories (these people seem to need an hour of running to burn off one potato chip).

Although the first group must grapple with putting on weight (and that's not as pretty a picture as it may seem), the second group is the dieting majority, whose dream is to raise their metabolisms, and so burn more calories for the buck.

"'How do I lose weight?' is asked a million different ways," says Kristin Reimers, M.S., R.D., associate director of the International Center for Sports Nutrition at the University of Nebraska Medical Center in Omaha. "The message that calories in to calories out equals weight loss has to come through loud and clear."

What Affects Your Metabolism?

Many factors affect metabolism, from body-fat ratio and hormone production to physical stress and age. Some are genetically determined, some are environmental, and some we can influence ourselves.

• **Body composition.** The bigger, the heavier, the more muscular you are, the higher your metabolic rate will be. The simple explanation: The heavier the body, the more energy it takes to move it around. A more complicated version: Resting metabolic rate is directly related to the body's total amount of metabolically active fat-free mass—all the parts, including muscle, bone, and organs, that aren't composed of less metabolically active fat. The more fat-free mass, the higher the metabolism, and bigger, heavier people have more such mass (even if it's hidden under layers of fat) than their smaller, leaner counterparts.

• **Body type.** The body type with which you're born affects your body composition, which affects metabolism. Muscular mesomorphs have a higher

Fluids Equal Fuel

Here are the fluid-intake recommendations for athletes:

Two hours
before activity . . . . 2 cups

Ten to fifteen minutes
before activity . . . . 2½ cups

Every fifteen minutes
during activity . . . . ½–¾ cup

After activity . . . . 2 cups
for every
pound lost

Source: American Dietetic Association

metabolic rate than slim ectomorphs. So do rounder, heavier endomorphs (and those who are overweight)—not because these people have a higher percentage of muscle, but because they simply have more of it.

• **Nerves and hormones.** The nervous system can stimulate the endocrine system to release hormones that speed or slow the metabolism, while hormones can prompt or block activity within the nerves. Emotional and physical stress, drugs, and diet all play a part here.

• **Vitamins and minerals.** A proper diet is crucial to support the chemical reactions and mechanisms needed for the body to metabolize food into energy.

• **Temperature.** When the body has to work to stay cool or warm, metabolic rates go up.

• **Drugs and stimulants.** The effect of certain drugs—caffeine, amphetamines, several hormones, even nicotine—on the nervous system can cause a temporary increase in metabolic rate. But side effects—including increases in heart rate and blood pressure—can be dangerous, and the overall effect on normal energy metabolism can at times have the opposite result, slowing the metabolism down. Physical and psychological dependence, and increased tolerance levels, can also occur.

"There are certainly substances on the market that increase metabolic rate," says Kristin Reimers. "'Is it safe?' becomes the question."

The short answer, in most cases, is no.

• **Illness and infection.** The work of fighting infection and illness can increase resting energy expenditure by 10 to 40 percent. When you run a fever, your basal metabolic rate will increase by 15 percent for each degree Celsius rise in body temperature.

• **Pregnancy.** Having a baby is a lot of work. The energy cost of pregnancy has been estimated at an average of 300 calories per day.

• **Eating and digestion.** Breaking down, digesting, and absorbing food takes energy. A healthy breakfast can temporarily boost resting metabolism by 10 percent or more.

• **Gender and age.** Women, who have more built-in body fat and less lean tissue than men, tend to have metabolisms 5 to 10 percent lower. The elderly, with decreasing levels of muscle mass, due in part to lower levels of activity, will experience a steady decline in metabolic rate.

Exercise and Metabolism

Bigger, heavier, more muscular people generally have higher metabolic rates. But while you can't get taller and don't want to get fatter, getting more muscular is both desirable and well within reach, thanks to the power of exercise.

"Fat is inactive tissue, where muscle is a more metabolically active tissue that burns more calories," says Chris Rosenbloom. "One of the big pluses of exercise is you can put on more muscle mass and so you can burn more calories throughout the day."

Even at rest, muscle tissue is busy burning

SMART MONEY

"Diets with an all-or-nothing approach, a reliance on supplements, or extreme altered eating habits—*only* protein, *no* carbohydrates, *no* fats, *no* liquids, *only* liquids—should be red flags," says Leslie Bonci, of the ADA.

Fad diets can be dangerous, and they rarely have a permanent effect. Very-low-calorie diets will backfire, too: Convinced it's starving, the body slows its metabolism to conserve energy. With "yo-yo dieting," where weight is gained and lost in cycles on severe, restricted diets, the metabolism falls lower and lower, and the extra weight actually increases and is harder to lose permanently.

Your best bet: Control calories in by eating healthy, low-fat foods; and stick with an exercise program you enjoy.

calories. Studies have found that increases in muscle mass from as few as three months of a moderate weight-training or resistance-training program can boost your resting metabolic rate. And even a small boost of your resting metabolic rate can significantly increase the rate at which calories are burned during activity.

Physical activity and exercise are the keys to the greatest change in energy metabolism by far. In just a few seconds of intense activity, muscles will use an amazing amount of energy. Sixty minutes of brisk walking or slow jogging can increase your energy expenditure ten-fold for that hour. High-intensity aerobic interval training has a major effect on your calorie-burning rate.

If that's not enough to convince you, there's a bonus called afterburn: a metabolic rate that stays elevated for as long as several hours after moderate to vigorous exercise. (Note: Afterburn following aerobic exercise does not last as long as afterburn following resistance training.)

The Great Food Pyramid

Three out of four Americans surveyed in an ADA/International Food Information Council survey said there's too much conflicting information about diet. No wonder. While once upon a time there were the four basic food groups, along came the more detailed USDA Food Guide Pyramid, to guard against not only our nutritional deficiencies but our excesses as well. The government's seven *Dietary Guidelines for Americans* are as follows:

• Eat a variety of foods.

• Balance the food you eat with physical activity— maintain or improve your weight.

• Choose a diet with plenty of grain products, vegetables, and fruits.

• Choose a diet low in fat, saturated fat, and cholesterol.

• Choose a diet moderate in sugars.

• Choose a diet moderate in salt and sodium.

• If you drink alcoholic beverages, do so in moderation.

Based on the U.S. Recommended Dietary Allowances (RDAs) for protein, vitamins, minerals, and dietary fiber, with emphasis on avoiding excessive amounts of calories, fat, saturated fat, cholesterol, sodium, sugars, and alcohol, the USDA Food Guide Pyramid was developed to help healthy Americans remain in good health by eating the right things in the right amounts. Follow its serving guidelines, and you'll get the right proportion of RDAs in every category you need—without having to count all those calories and grams.

Okay. We can handle that. But then came the Mediterranean pyramid, the Asian pyramid, and the Latin American pyramid, developed by Oldways Preservation and Exchange Trust to point us toward diets of cultures linked with good health. And then the Puerto Rican pyramid, the Vegetarian pyramid, and the Soul Food pyramid, which use the USDA pyramid framework with a tailored range of foods.

F.Y.I.

What we believe and do:
The percentage of Americans who:

Believe nutrition
impacts health 79

Are doing all they
can to achieve a
healthful eating
plan. 39

Skip meals "very
often" or "quite
a bit" 28

Believe it's
necessary to
take a nutrition
supplement to
ensure proper
health 35

Think they need
to eliminate all
fat from their
diets 13

Believe foods
are either "good"
or "bad" 72

*Source: American Dietetic
Association 1997 Nutrition
Trends Survey*

By now it's more confusing than the Riddle of the Sphinx.

"The message is there's no one ideal diet," says Kristin Reimers. "Most people can improve their diet by doing simple things, like adding more fruits and vegetables, and cutting back on fats . . . but not at the expense of cutting out [all] dairy and meats. Can you get a balanced diet without them? Sure." But take their absence into account.

"The other pyramids are alternatives and give food for thought," says Kristine Clark, Ph.D., R.D., director of sports nutrition at the Center for Sports Medicine at Penn State University, "but the basic food group pyramid is a high-quality tool. It predominately teaches portion control—the message the consumer pays least attention to. The exerciser thinks he can eat all the carbohydrates he wants, or all the fat-free foods he wants. That's a huge misconception."

One of the biggest food myths is that foods are either good or bad. The truth: All kinds of foods are good for us—as long as we eat a good balance of all kinds of foods.

If you don't eat any food from one or more of the groups, be sure you're nutritionally covered. If you're lactose intolerant, for example, replace milk with yogurt or cheese (calcium-fortified juices or supplements provide only one of several nutrients contained in the dairy group). If you exclude red meats, find other sources of zinc. Vegans, who eat no animal, egg, or dairy products, can get their protein requirements from legumes, nuts, and seeds in combination with whole-grain breads and cereals. For athletes, the volume of vegetarian foods required to meet energy needs is greater than the stomach can hold; several smaller meals through the day is a good idea.

Remember, the goal of the food pyramids is to help you to eat for health.

"People become confused because we try to interject all kinds of nutrition principles into one big pot," says Reimers. "It's important not to mix messages based on performance with weight loss."

Eating to lose weight is a calories in/calories out equation. Eating for health is where high fiber, low fat, and lots of fruits and vegetables come in (though, of course, the healthier your body, the better able it is to process those calories).

Building the Pyramid for You

Depending on your gender, age, and level of physical activity, you'll have different caloric needs, and different amounts of daily servings appropriate for you. The USDA offers some general daily guidelines: 1,600 calories have been estimated to be "about right" for many sedentary women and some older adults; 2,200 calories for most children, teenage girls, active women (women who are pregnant or lactating may need somewhat more), and many sedentary men; and 2,800 calories for teenage boys, many active men, and some very active women.

Another method: Multiply your body weight in pounds by whichever of the following numbers applies:

Activity Level	Male	Female
Light	17	16
Moderate	19	17
Heavy	23	20

F.Y.I.

Why we don't eat well: The percentage of Americans who:

Fear giving up foods 40

Are confused or frustrated over nutrition studies/reports . . . 23

Believe that a healthful eating style takes too much time 21

Source: American Dietetic Association 1997 Nutrition Trends Survey

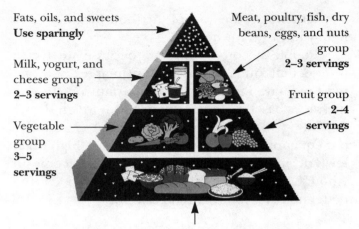

Fats, oils, and sweets
Use sparingly

Meat, poultry, fish, dry beans, eggs, and nuts group
2–3 servings

Milk, yogurt, and cheese group
2–3 servings

Fruit group
2–4 servings

Vegetable group
3–5 servings

Bread, cereal, rice, and pasta group **6–11 servings**

Then follow USDA recommendations for number of servings for the different food groups. For example:

	1,600 calories	2,200 calories	2,800 calories
Bread group servings	6	9	11
Fruit group servings	2	3	4
Vegetable group servings	3	4	5
Meat group (daily total)	5 oz.	6 oz.	7 oz.
Milk group servings	2–3*	2–3*	2–3*
Total fat (grams) **	53	73	93
Total added sugars *(teaspoons)* **	6	12	18

* Women who are pregnant or lactating, teenagers, and young adults to age twenty-four need three servings.

** Including fat and added sugars from all food choices.

Portion Size Counts

It's smart to read a label to learn that one serving of fat-free chocolate fudge ice cream contains 100 calories before you eat it. It's not so smart to expect that same (half-cup) calorie count when you fill a big bowl to the brim.

The serving sizes in the USDA Food Guide Pyramid and on food labels serve different purposes. Here are some examples of one serving as defined by the pyramid.

Bread, cereal, rice, pasta

1 slice of bread
1 small roll, biscuit, or muffin
5 to 6 small crackers
1/2 cup cooked cereal, rice, or pasta
1 ounce ready-to-eat cereal

Fruits

1 medium fruit such as an apple or banana
½ grapefruit
¾ cup juice
½ cup berries
½ cup canned fruit
¼ cup dried fruit

Vegetables

½ cup cooked or chopped raw vegetables
1 cup leafy raw vegetables such as lettuce, Swiss chard, or spinach
¾ cup vegetable juice

Meats, poultry, fish, dry beans and peas, eggs, nuts

2–3 ounces of cooked lean meat, poultry without skin, or fish

STREET SMARTS

"Healthy snacks during the day keep me from gorging at mealtime, and knowing I can eat a little bit later takes the pressure off my need to clean the plate," says fifty-two-year-old accountant Anne Arnon, who successfully lost more than twenty pounds and has kept it off for more than a year. "Smaller dishes and silverware also make portions look bigger," she says. "They may be mind games, but they really help."

4 ounces tofu
Count 1 egg, ½ cup cooked beans, or 2 table-spoons peanut butter as 1 ounce of meat

Milk, yogurt, cheese
1 cup milk
8 ounces yogurt
2 ounces processed cheese

Fats, oils, sweets, alcoholic beverages
Use fats and sweets sparingly.
Drink alcohol in moderation, if at all.

Note: The food pyramid doesn't differentiate high-fat foods from healthier choices, so read labels and watch what you take in.

The ADA's *Complete Food and Nutrition Guide* gives some rules of thumb for determining portion sizes when your measuring cup or scale aren't around:

• Three ounces of meat, poultry, or fish are about the size of a deck of playing cards.

• One-half cup of fruit, vegetables, pasta, or rice is about the size of a small fist.

• One ounce of cheese is about the size of your thumb.

• One cup of milk, yogurt, or chopped fresh greens is about the size of a small hand holding a tennis ball.

Fats: Not Necessarily Evil

Life would be much simpler if all fats were bad, but it wouldn't be as tasty, and it wouldn't be nutritionally complete. Just as we need some body fat to be healthy and perform at optimal levels, we need some dietary fat (the kind found in foods) to be healthy, too. Among other benefits, it allows us to absorb and use fat-soluble vitamins like A, D, E, and K, and it helps us feel full longer so we don't overeat. Linoleic acid, a type of fat that can be supplied only by the foods we eat, is necessary for growth and reproduction, and helps protect us from excessive loss of water and damage from the sun's ultraviolet rays.

Some fats are better for us than others. Studies have linked an increase in saturated fats with a harmful increase in blood cholesterol levels (see "Cholesterol: The Good and the Bad," page 129) and an increased risk of heart attack. But when unsaturated fats or oils (particularly the monoun-saturated type) replace saturated fat, the amount of blood cholesterol—and heart disease risk—goes down.

Good news/bad news: All fats—no matter what kind—contain nine calories per gram, more than twice as many calories as carbohydrates or protein. This concentrated source of energy can be helpful for extremely active types who couldn't otherwise get enough calories without consuming massive quantities of food, but for the ordinary human, the excess calories can lead to unwanted weight gain.

Overall, however, all fats should be kept at low

SMART DEFINITIONS

Olestra
Known also by its brand name, Olean, this no-fat "fat replacer" is a synthetic mixture of sugar and vegetable oil. Because its molecules are much larger than those of ordinary fats, the body's digestive enzymes cannot break them down and olestra is not absorbed when eaten—it travels through the body and straight out, like high-fiber bran (and it might take some vitamins and nutrients along with it). It might also have the similar get-me-to-the-bathroom effect.

levels for good health. The American Heart Association (AHA) recommends that our diet contain no more than 30 percent of its total calories from fat—only 10 percent of that from saturated fat, 10 percent from polyunsaturated fat, and 10 percent from monounsaturated fat. To figure that out, multiply your caloric intake by .10 and divide by 9, the number of calories in each gram of fat. Food labels differentiate saturated fat content from the overall amount of fat contained.

Remember, reduced-fat foods are not always low in fat, they just contain less of it. And neither are fat-free or lower-fat foods the sole answer to staying slim. They still contain calories. "We call it 'the SnackWell's Cookie Syndrome'—that I can eat the whole box," says Kristine Clark. "Nothing could be farther from the truth." To lose weight, you need to take in less energy (fewer calories) than you work off.

The Bad, the Better, and Somewhere in Between

Although we differentiate between "saturated" and "unsaturated," all fats contain a mixture of both kinds of fatty acids—fat building blocks—with the type that predominates determining what we call it.

• **The bad fats.** Saturated fats, like butter and lard, generally are solid at room temperature. The tropical vegetable oils palm, palm kernel, and coconut also contain higher levels of saturated fats.

• **The better fats.** Unsaturated fats—polyunsaturated and monounsaturated—like olive, canola, safflower, sunflower, soybean, corn, and other vegetable oils, are liquid at room temperature.

• **Somewhere in the middle.** Trans fats occur naturally in meat and dairy products and in processed foods that are hydrogenated, (in which liquid vegetable oils are converted into more solid forms, such as solid shortening and stick margarine). Although not quite as harmful as saturated fats, trans fats have been compared with saturated fats in terms of their effect on blood cholesterol. The FDA currently requires only total fat and saturated fats be listed on the food label; look for "partially hydrogenated" vegetable oil.

Cholesterol: The Good and the Bad

Blood cholesterol is an important chemical found in blood, tissue, and the body's digestive juices. Dietary cholesterol is found in some of the foods we eat, and may have little effect on the amount of cholesterol in the blood. The body produces about 80 percent of its blood cholesterol, mostly determined by genetics, the total amount of fat, and the type of fat that is eaten, not how much cholesterol we consume. One tablespoon of a popular brand of corn oil, for instance, contains no cholesterol but will affect our blood cholesterol level with its 2 grams of saturated fat, 8 grams of polyunsaturated fat, and 3.5 grams of monounsaturated fat. Again, to reduce elevated blood cholesterol levels, the AHA recommends restricting dietary fat.

SMART SOURCES

Center for Nutrition Policy and Promotion 1120 20th St., N.W. Suite 200, North Lobby Washington, DC 20036 202-606-8000 www.usda.gov/fcs/cnpp.htm

This organization of the U.S. Department of Agriculture Food Information Council provides a link between consumer, nutrition educator, and scientific research. Write or visit the web site for its publication, *Nutrition Insights,* or copies of the USDA Food Guide Pyramid and *Dietary Guidelines for Americans.*

In the body, cholesterol is involved in the creation of lipoproteins: LDL (low-density lipoproteins) and HDL (high-density lipoproteins). LDL (known as the "bad" cholesterol") blocks the walls of the arteriesand leads to heart disease. HDL (the "good" cholesterol) can remove the LDL and counteract its harmful effects. When your doctor gives you your cholesterol level, the LDL/HDL ratio is a significant thing to know.

This is where our fat intake matters so much. Saturated fats are linked with an increase in "bad" LDL and its health risks, while unsaturated fats are linked with a decrease in the harmful stuff. The thing is, polyunsaturated fats have also been linked with a decrease in "good" HDL; only monounsaturated fats, such as olive and canola oils, and nuts, decrease LDL while leaving untouched or slightly raising its beneficial counterpart.

But don't overlook the genetic component. "In some people, a low-fat diet may even have a negative effect on their cholesterol profile," says Kristin Reimers. "While we used to think 'one size fits all,' that's no longer true. The message for today is probably for most people, the recommendation of 30 percent of calories from fat is appropriate, but if they discover that their cholesterol profile is out of whack, they need to be careful."

Carbohydrates: Energy to Go

Carbohydrates are the most readily available—and the body's preferred—source of food energy, and for someone who's working out, they're like high-test in the tank. Glycogen, a substance produced by the body and stored in the muscles and liver—and the energy source on which working muscles draw—can be manufactured only from dietary carbohydrates and isn't stored in great quantity, so it's crucial to keep the carbohydrates coming in if you're working out.

How much carbohydrate you need each day to replace muscle glycogen depends on your size. One rule of thumb: Eat five to six grams of carbohydrate per kilogram you weigh. (To convert your body weight into kilograms, divide your weight in pounds by 2.2.) That should translate into about 55 to 60 percent of your daily caloric intake.

Complex Carbohydrates, Simple Carbohydrates

Not just in bread and pasta, carbohydrates come from a wide variety of sources, and in several forms. Complex carbohydrates—starches and dietary fiber, found in potatoes, rice, pasta, some vegetables, bread, and cereal—consist of long chains of sugar molecules and tend to be low in calories and fat, high in fiber, and take some time for the body to break down. In this gradual process, your blood-sugar level and energy remain fairly constant, leaving you feeling full for a comfortable period of time.

Sugars—not just the kind you borrow from your neighbor, but including the lactose in milk products and the fructose in fruits—are simple carbohydrates, one- or two-molecule combinations that are absorbed quickly and cause blood-sugar levels to leap and then drop, often to a level

SMART SOURCES

Center for Science in the Public Interest
1875 Connecticut Ave., N.W.
Suite 300
Washington, DC 20009
202-332-9110
www.cspinet.org

The mission of this nonprofit education and advocacy organization: "Improving the safety and nutritional quality of our food supply and . . . reducing the carnage caused by alcoholic beverages." One of the ways it does so is by educating the public. Their *Nutrition Action Healthletter* offers some very helpful and entertainingly written advice.

Carbo Loading

Remember when marathoners would spend days before an event gorging on pasta and we'd all wish we were runners, too? While it may be helpful for high-intensity endurance sports requiring ninety minutes or more of nonstop action, if you're eating the recommended 55 to 60 percent of your diet in carbohydrates daily, there's no need—or excuse—to "load" carbohydrates or the glycogen they contain. Your muscles always have enough. In the same vein, watch out for energy bars, designed for the very active person and not for people doing aerobics three times a week. "Energy is just another name for calories," says Chris Rosenbloom, who calls them "glorified candy bars." "You can gain weight from taking in too much."

below where they started. Sugar highs and lows can leave you feeling drained and hungry again.

For very active people with very high calorie needs, sugars can be a quick source of energy. Most of us aren't that active, though, and are better off with carbohydrates of the complex kind. Beside their harmful impact on tooth decay and mood swings, sugar-heavy foods tend to supply calories but few or no nutrients and should be used in moderation by most healthy people, and sparingly by those who need to watch their weight.

Better sources of sugars are those that don't involve the white, powdery type. Good sources of complex carbohydrates include whole-grain breads, enriched rice and pasta, and oatmeal.

During digestion all carbohydrates except fiber break down into sugars. Soluble fiber, found in oats, beans, and soy-based foods, is broken down in the intestines; insoluble fiber, such as that found in wheat bran, just passes right through the digestive tract, and out. Found only in plant foods, fiber can not only help you feel fuller but has been linked with lower rates of heart disease, colon cancer, and diabetes, and the soluble kind has been linked with lowered cholesterol.

Some caveats: Increased levels of fiber can give you, shall we say, quite a workout in the bathroom, so add fiber to your diet gradually to allow your body to adjust. At very high levels, some high-fiber foods, such as wheat bran, can interfere with mineral absorption, so avoid fiber concentrates in favor of mineral-containing foods. Increased consumption of fiber should be accompanied by an increased intake of water, too.

Good sources of fiber include bran, barley, lentils, peas and beans, apples, citrus fruits, and carrots.

Vitamins, Minerals, and Supplements

Approximately 3,400 different vitamin and mineral products are available to consumers, for which we spend $4 billion a year, according to the ADA. Do we need them? It all depends on what we eat. A well-balanced, nutritious diet based on the Food Guide Pyramid principles will more than satisfy the RDAs for vitamins and minerals, but many people take a multivitamin-mineral supplement as "insurance."

There are some dangers. Dietary supplements are not required to prove safety and efficacy, so the buyer should beware. Also, megadoses of single-nutrient supplements can lead to harmful levels of some vitamins and minerals (vitamins A and D produce well-defined toxic syndromes, and even water-soluble vitamins like niacin and vitamin B6 can cause adverse effects when taken in large amounts) or block the effect of others you need. Large doses of iron, for instance, can cause an iron toxicity and influence the body's absorption of magnesium and zinc. Excessive doses of vitamins are conventionally defined as around ten or more times the RDA, but toxic effects from

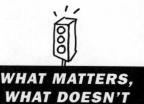

WHAT MATTERS, WHAT DOESN'T

What Matters

• A balanced diet, low in fats and high in healthy carbohydrates.

• Plenty of fluids.

• Food that tastes good, to keep you eating right.

• Portion size.

What Doesn't

• One food to the exclusion of all others.

• Power-in-a-can products or energy bars.

• Megadoses of diet supplements or vitamins.

• Cutting out all fats.

• Miracle claims from people without an R.D. (registered dietitian) after their names.

long-term ingestion of, for instance, vitamin A has been documented with supplements of only five times the RDA. Too much protein will be stored as fat; imbalanced amino acid diets associated with protein supplements are associated with depressed growth.

Absorption is another issue. Many vitamins contain more of a substance than the body can process at a time. The result is what Victor Herbert, M.D., coauthor of *The Vitamin Pushers,* calls "expensive urine." Four billion dollars' worth.

Protein: Fallen Hero

Remember when protein was the all-American health hero? No more. Most of us eat far too much of it, often in the form of fat-heavy meats and cheese. That doesn't mean we don't need to take in any, of course—nine of the many amino acids of which proteins are composed (called essential amino acids) can be garnered only through food.

Protein is not the primary source of energy so many people credit it to be (weight-lifters taking protein supplements, take note). Its main functions are to maintain and repair muscle and other tissues; make hemoglobin, which carries oxygen to exercising muscles; form antibodies to fight infection and

A Sugar by Any Other Name

If you don't see the word "sugar" on a food label, that doesn't mean it isn't there. Here are some of the most common. If one of them is the first or second item on the ingredients list, or several appear, watch out.

- Corn sweetener
- Dextrose
- Fructose
- Fruit juice concentrate
- Glucose
- Honey
- Lactose
- Maltose
- Molasses
- Sucrose
- Syrup

disease; and produce enzymes and hormones that regulate body processes. When carbohydrates and fats aren't consumed in sufficient supply for energy needs, the body will turn to protein as a last resort.

The RDA for proteins is .6 grams per kilogram of weight (divide your weight in pounds by 2.2 and multiply by .6), slightly more for women who are pregnant or lactating, the elderly, children, and young adults. Too little and your body can't properly function. Too much and the amino acids are stored as fat.

Good sources of protein include milk and yogurt, cooked legumes like beans and peas, and lean meat, fish, and poultry. Whenever possible, consume your proteins in the healthiest way you can: Fat-free cottage cheese, for instance, offers 13 grams per one-half cup, without any fat at all.

Water: Drink It Everywhere

You can live longer without food than you can without water, second only to oxygen as essential to life. Muscular athletes may look solid, but they aren't: 70 percent of those bodies are made up of the liquid stuff.

Like many machines, the body produces heat when it's working, and constantly cools itself by releasing water via our lungs and skin. The more physically active you are, the harder you're working your body, the more water you lose (a 150-pound athlete can sweat as much as six cups in one hour). If that water isn't replaced, dehydra-

THE BOTTOM LINE

A balanced eating plan that supplies the right amount of nutrients and energy through a wide variety of foods is essential for staying on track and in good health. People on exercise programs especially need to supply their bodies with adequate fluids and plenty of low-fat, high-carbohydrate foods that fuel the energy requirements of physical activity, paying careful attention to nutrition needs before, during, and after exercise. For weight loss, regular physical activity and reduced calories are the keys; "miracle" products, severely restricted diets, and one-dimensional approaches don't work.

tion can follow, with its accompanying decrease in endurance and increased risk of serious heat exhaustion and heat stroke.

"There's a Catch-22 because the body is needing more but the sensation of thirst is diminishing," says the ADA's Leslie Bonci. "So it's absolutely critical that you train yourself to drink. You see people exercising in the heat and pouring the water over them. I tell them it has to go *in* to do the job."

Before, during, and after exercise, for most athletes, water is best. Diluted fruit juices and fruit drinks can help maintain the body's energy supply while replenishing lost fluids, but when they're taken full-strength, the sugar they contain can cause bloating and cramps.

All those sports drinks on the market? The idea is that electrolytes and carbohydrates help you absorb fluid more readily into the bloodstream and replace minerals you lose in sweat. But many contain stimulants like ephedra and caffeine, which can dehydrate you. And while small amounts of sugar can enhance water absorption and, for prolonged, intense activities, delay muscle fatigue, too much sugar can have the opposite effect.

"The research shows that anybody who's exercising for less than an hour at a time just needs water," says Chris Rosenbloom, adding a special note for those concerned about their weight. "Be careful about adding extra calories in fluids that more than make up for what you're using up during exercise."

The one benefit of those sports drinks: the taste. The more you like something, the more you'll down. Mix a little bit of sugar or fruit juice into your water and you'll have a healthier, less expensive drink.

CHAPTER 7

Other Roads to Fitness

It's often thought of as "New Age," but a lot of it has been around for thousands of years. "Alternative," "Eastern," or "integrative" medicine—whatever you choose to call it—has been used to cure everything from colds to cancer. And many of these unconventional approaches to medicine can be adopted in a fitness program to enhance performance, increase flexibility, ease the pain of workout-related injury, and improve well-being overall.

What Exactly Is Alternative?

What is alternative? The short answer is, any treatment or health-care practice not generally taught in medical schools, not generally used in hospitals, and not generally covered by medical insurance. But more and more medical schools, hospitals, and insurance policies are broadening their view.

"There's a paradigm shift going on in American health care toward alternative medicine," says Jerome F. McAndrews, D.C., national spokesperson for the American Chiropractic Association and a member of the advisory board of the American Association of Alternative Medicine, an organization out to fill the void in communication between alternative health-care systems and the public.

No longer content to confine health care to established Western ways, Americans have started to investigate a broader range of medical methods.

A major eye-opener occurred in January 1993, when Harvard physician David Eisenberg, Ph.D., M.D., published a landmark survey in the *New England Journal of Medicine.* In 1990, the year of his study, Americans made 388 million visits to primary-care physicians . . . but saw alternative-care providers such as chiropractors, acupuncturists, and massage therapists 37 million times more. And, in the great majority of instances, they paid out of their own pockets, at that.

Today, the National Institutes of Health (NIH) includes an Office of Alternative Medicine; 3,000 conventionally trained American physicians have taken courses to incorporate acupuncture into their medical practices; at least 50 of the 125 medical schools in the United States now offer classes in unconventional therapies; and even the health insurance industry has begun to take note—and issue coverage—with NIH blessings.

"People are open to it more than ever," says Dahelia Hunt, director of professional fitness instructor training at the Baylor Sports Medicine Institute in Houston, who's seeing increasing interest in the stress-management aspects of alternative health care, from massage to movement therapies to seeking the spiritual in one's self— "anything that doesn't pound the body any more."

Just as any one exercise may provide greater or lesser degrees of both aerobic and anaerobic training, less conventional approaches often fall into more than one category or field. The Pilates Method, for instance, described in chapter 3, takes a mind-body approach to improving body flexibility and strength. Yoga encompasses a philosophy of being that goes far beyond a methodology for twisting yourself into a pretzel shape.

Then, of course, some are less conventional

SMART SOURCES

Alternative Health

Office of Alternative Medicine Clearinghouse
National Institutes of Health
P.O. Box 8218
Silver Spring, MD 20907
888-644-6226
http://altmed.od.nih.gov/

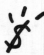

SMART MONEY

"In America, we think if a little is good, more is better," says fitness professional Dahelia Hunt of the Baylor Sports Medicine Institute. "We're the only society in the world that overexercises. We're abusing our bodies constantly with fitness, fitness, fitness."

Massage, spiritual renewal, touch and movement therapies, and other "alternative" techniques can help provide the rest and relaxation that are important components of a healthy fitness plan.

than others: A massage therapist might be relatively easy to find; a Feldenkrais practitioner might require a bit more searching.

Most of these approaches are not intended to exclude but to complement others, of both the conventional and nonconventional sort. Reputable practitioners won't espouse an "I'm all you need" philosophy any more than a doctor would tell you not to go to a dentist. Remember, seeing a chiropractor for your low-back pain can be very helpful, but it doesn't mean you shouldn't know where the hospital emergency room is.

The Mind-Body Connection

Back when the dangers we faced came from lions and tigers, our minds helped protect our bodies by calling for a surge of adrenaline. Our hearts would beat faster, our blood pressure would rise, and our breath would come hard and fast, providing the burst of energy we'd need for escape. Today, when psychological stress is our greatest enemy, we still experience this "fight or flight" response—about fifty times a day, says Alice D. Domar, Ph.D., author of *Healing Mind, Healthy Woman,* with the Mind/Body Medical Institute at Beth Israel Deaconess Medical Center and Harvard Medical School's Division of Behavioral Medicine. "It's almost like your body goes into overdrive, and that can lead to an enormous list of physical symptoms"—hypertension, insomnia, migraine, and more.

The flip side to all this potential damage: What goes on in our minds can help us as well.

According to the Mind/Body Medical Institute, studies have proven the effects of "behavioral medicine interventions," relaxation techniques like meditation, imagery, prayer, and deep breathing—in addition to good nutrition and moderate exercise—on everything from infertility to chronic pain.

Hypnosis

Used to treat everything from eating disorders to migraines, hypnosis has been praised as a pain-fighter in the *Journal of the American Medical Association* and has long been relied upon for all manner of stress relief. In contrast to the zombie-like trance we see in movie portrayals, hypnosis is a comfortable state of deep relaxation. And you don't have to lose consciousness for it to work.

"The idea that someone is doing something *to* you, that you're somehow under this person's spell—this is the fear," says Joan S. Ingalls, Ed.D., who has a private consulting practice in sports mental training in Portsmouth, New Hampshire. "Hypnosis can only happen if the person who is the subject wants to go into hypnosis and that person actually puts himself into a trance. That person can still choose to do what he chooses to do or not to."

Athletes use hypnotherapeutic techniques (either hypnosis or self-hypnosis) to build confidence, reinforce goals, motivate and energize, and deal with performance fears. To eliminate the mental aspect of fatigue, Ingalls, a mental-training consultant to the Durham Boat Club, has helped rowers learn what might be called productive forgetfulness: After every twenty-one strokes rowed,

SMART SOURCES

Hypnosis

The Milton H. Erickson
  Foundation
3606 N. 24th St.
Phoenix, AZ 85016
602-956-6196
www.erickson
foundation.org

they'd "forget" the first twenty and feel like they were starting out on stroke one. "This is a neat little trick to stay feeling fresh throughout a race or even a workout," says Ingalls.

The monotonous, repetitive movement of many longer-length exercise routines has built-in potential for inducing hypnotic trance. (If you've ever been walking along on the treadmill and been surprised by the cool-down beeper after what seems like you just began, congratulations: You've been there.) The state of mind can be productive in more ways than one.

"By concentrating on monitoring all the physiological adaptations to the exercise," such as breathing patterns, muscle response, and so on, says Ingalls, "a person who's open and receptive can shift into a kind of trance state. The exercise period can double as a meditation time, and when the workout is over, you feel rejuvenated and refreshed."

Biofeedback

Biofeedback operates on the premise that by becoming aware of internal, involuntary bodily functions (from brain activity to muscle tension to pulse rate to stress level and others), we can bring them under our control, and improve our health and our performance as well.

With a biofeedback monitor providing auditory or visual information about what's going on inside us, we can get a handle on physical reactions and processes that were formerly thought to be beyond our reach. For instance, a monitor might sound a beeper or flash a light whenever your muscles tense. To relax the muscles, you would need to slow down the beeping, which sounds like putting the cart before the horse, but, nevertheless, has been proved to work. In the process, we learn to associate sensations from the muscle with actual levels of tension, and so learn how to relax them on demand. And no, you don't need to stay "hooked up" forever: After biofeedback treatment in study group populations, people were able to repeat their response with no sensors attached.

Biofeedback techniques have been used to treat a long list of conditions, including muscle spasms, muscle dysfunction caused by injury, chronic pain, movement disorders, headache, and many other afflictions of body and mind. Its place in sports? The director of the Princeton Biofeedback Centre in New Jersey, Lester G. Fehmi, Ph.D., served as a biofeedback and attention-training consultant to the Dallas Cowboys and New Jersey Nets.

Meditation and Prayer

From deep breathing to creative visualization; with the aid of a mantra or by a candle's flame; done in conjunction with physical movement or by confining the "motion" to the mind—for countless years, meditation and prayer have been bringing their adherents a sense of peace they hardly needed science to verify.

Researchers now believe the medical impact of meditation may connect with its effects on cortisol, a hormone released by the body in response to stress. While cortisol is helpful during occasional "fight or flight" situations, its continual release in response to the daily stresses of modern life can inhibit the immune system and slow tissue repair. Meditation may slow or reverse this process. In studies, people taught transcendental meditation (TM) had cortisol levels 15 percent lower than before they had become meditators. Another study found that long-term meditators had a drop in cortisol levels of nearly 25 percent.

Harvard Medical School's Herbert Benson, M.D., calls it the "relaxation response" and offers training in the method at the Mind/Body Institute and Division of Behavioral Medicine, of which he is the director. The eminent physician, researcher, and best-selling author, who believes we're nourished by meditation and prayer, emotional expression and support, reports benefits in everything from PMS to HIV.

Religious belief and faith are prompting "amens" from the scientific community as well.

"I'm not saying that physicians should supplant clergy or that prayer should supplant Prozac," said Dr. Dale A. Matthews, a researcher at Georgetown University, as quoted in *USA Today.* But Matthews does "believe that physicians can and should encourage patients' autonomous religious activities."

At the 1997 meeting of the American Association for the Advancement of Science, Matthews and other researchers presented evidence of the positive influence of religious belief on health. A review of 212 studies found three out of four showing benefits.

One theory: Like meditation, prayer and ritual might slow the production of harmful stress hormones in the body. Studies have shown this kind of stress reduction can reduce high blood pressure, chronic pain, insomnia, and infertility, among other ills.

Then there are other possibilities: One San Francisco study randomly divided 393 seriously ill heart patients into two groups. Half were prayed for, half were not; the individuals did not know which group they were in. The prayer recipients suffered fewer health complications. Praise the Lord.

Yoga

By now a familiar class at the health club, yoga is more than a set of physical positions and breathing techniques; it is a meditative approach and a way of life that promotes a more limber physical and mental state. Along with improved flexibility and muscle tone, yoga can offer the stress-reducing, bodily-function-controlling, disease-risk-lowering benefits of other mind-body techniques.

From the Sanskrit root *yuj* or *yui,* meaning to yoke, as animals are yoked to combine their strength and channel their direction, yoga in the true sense combines a belief system, diet, and exercise to integrate spirit, body, and mind. But you don't have to be a total convert to reap benefits of the life philosophy.

You don't have to be a contortionist, either; beginner-level classes and different yoga styles can accommodate every body's level. There are several popular types of hatha yoga, the sort that's related to physical exercise (as opposed to the sexually oriented tantra yoga, which you probably won't find offered in classes at the local gym). Ashtanga, Sanskrit for "eight limbs," refers to the eight aspects of yoga and at times has been offered as sort of the circuit training of the yoga world, with rapid transition from one posture to the next to promote strength, stamina, and bodywide

STREET SMARTS

"I remember when massage was a great treat I'd enjoy on vacation, but it's become a life-saver when my migraines take hold," says Nancy Tudor, a forty-one-year-old full-time mom. The difference between Swedish and neuro-muscular approaches can mean the difference between almost recreational relaxation and therapeutic cure.

movement of heat. Iyengar yoga is more static, with a focus on precise body alignment and positioning. Gentle yoga, flow yoga, and power yoga are a few Americanized versions you'll find.

In Touch: Massage and Body Work

One of the most ancient types of health care, from diagnosis to healing, involves the laying on of hands. Many "touch therapies" or "manual healing" techniques—massage, body work, acupressure, and the like—are based on a similar set of ideas:

• The concept of helping the body to heal itself, *vis medicatrix naturae*

• The conviction that stimulating one part of the body can affect other areas as well

• The belief that blockages or misalignments of bodily structure (be they from the effects of gravity, injury, conditions at birth, or repetitive movements of some kind) throw the body off kilter; bring the body back into alignment and it will return to health.

By loosening stiff, aching muscles, for instance, some massage therapists believe they can release "memories" of illness stored within; chiropractors manipulate the spine and skeletal structure to bring the body back into balance; and reflexologists "reach" numerous body organs and systems via areas of the feet and hands. Bio-Magnetic Touch Healing uses light touch (no magnets) on specific points on the body to activate our innate curative powers, much like acupressure, acupuncture, and shiatsu massage techniques.

Massage

Massage therapy, or therapeutic massage, is more than just a terrific way to relax. All that rubbing, kneading, pressing, and stroking has real health benefits, from improving circulation to speeding recovery from—or reducing the likelihood of—injury. Musculoskeletal, circulatory, and nervous systems all can benefit.

"A lot of people are using massage to aid in the recovery of injuries," says Beth Danner, of the National Certification Board for Therapeutic Massage and Body Work (NCBTMBW) in McLean, Virginia, who mentions pre- and postsurgical massage approaches, as well as on-site corporate facilities for employees to reduce stress. "The field is growing in the way that people use it, and in how often."

It's also growing in the number of massage therapists. More than thirty thousand are certified through NCBTMBW, and five hundred more are tested each month.

Although all forms of massage involve manipulation of soft body tissue (usually with the hands, but often with the forearms and elbows and sometimes with the feet), with the aim of returning the tissue to a healthy, normal state, there are a plethora of methods of approach. Here, some of the more common:

SMART SOURCES

Massage and Body Work

National Certification
   Board for Thera-
   peutic Massage and
   Body Work
8201 Greensboro Dr.
Suite 300
McLean, VA 22102
800-296-0664
703-610-9015
www.ncbtmb.com/

• **Aromatherapy.** More than just a good-smelling sensory experience, this infusion of herbal components into the massage oil is designed to offer a variety of effects, from invigorating, to toxin-relieving, to put-you-right-to-sleep.

• **Neuromuscular massage.** This populart therapeutic approach relies on circulation-stimulating pressure to break the stress-tension-pain cycle.

• **Shiatsu.** A Japanese massage technique using finger pressure on the body's meridian points, to affect channels of energy flow.

• **Sports massage.** Using elements from many types of body work, sports massage focuses on muscle systems that have to do with a particular sport. The goal: To improve performance, speed postevent recovery, and help muscle-related injuries heal.

• **Swedish massage.** This is the classic: long, deep, kneading strokes, combined with movement of the joints.

• **Trigger point and myotherapy.** These pain-relief techniques are used to relieve muscle spasms and cramping. Seven to ten seconds of pressure are applied to the trigger points—areas where muscles have been damaged and where blood flow is reduced—and then muscles are gently stretched.

Reflexology/Zone Therapy

No, it's not just foot massage. Reflexology traces its roots to ancient Indian, Chinese, and Egyptian civilization, and (like acupressure and shiatsu massage) is based on the idea that stimulating reflexes in one area of the body can affect corresponding body parts.

In 1913, American ear, nose, and throat physician Dr. William Fitzgerald introduced a version of reflexology to the West in which the body is considered to be made up of ten zones, with the hands and feet acting as "communication terminals."

Both reflexology and zone therapy operate on the same basic premise: Following illness, stress, injury, or disease, the body is in a state of "imbalance," and energy pathways are blocked. The hands of a trained practitioner can detect these problems and, by applying gentle pressure, release the blockages and restore the energy to its natural healthy flow.

Treatment sessions are often relaxing and pleasant enough to be confused with massage, and usually last about an hour. At times, however, fleeting discomfort, nausea, or even tearfulness might be proof positive of the elsewhere-based congestion or imbalance the reflexologist seeks. After all, who ever heard of nauseated feet?

Alphabet Soup of Certification

Acupuncture

Dipl. Ac.	Diploma in Acupuncture (NCCA certified)
D. Acu.	Doctor of Acupuncture (Occidental Institute Research Foundation)
L. Ac.	Licensed Acupuncturist
R. Ac.	Registered Acupuncturist

Chiropractic

D.C.	Doctor of Chiropractic

Massage Therapy

CMT	Certified Massage Therapist
LMT	Licensed Massage Therapist
CNMT	Certified Neuromuscular Therapist
LNMT	Licensed Neuromuscular Therapist

SMART SOURCES

Chiropractic

American Chiropractic
  Association
1701 Clarendon Blvd.
Arlington, VA 22209
800-986-INFO
703-276-8800

Chiropractic

In 1895, Daniel David Palmer delivered the first chiropractic adjustment to Harvey Lillard, a janitor in his office with an aching back. From that one adjustment, Lillard, who had been deaf since childhood, would experience a full recovery—back, hearing, and all.

They won't claim to restore hearing to the deaf, but the 55,000 licensed practitioners of chiropractic today in the United States make it the third largest doctoral-level health profession, after medicine and dentistry. Millions of Americans turn to chiropractors every year for conservative management of back pain, neck pain, and headaches without surgery or drugs. "Natural, hands-on health care," in the American Chiropractic Association's (ACA) words.

Where massage deals with the manipulation of soft tissue, chiropractic focuses on the relationship between skeletal structure (chiefly the spine) and function (the nervous system). By finding and treating structural problems that can affect the nervous system, in other words, they can put you in better shape. And the doctor of chiropractic's—or D.C.'s—preferred prescription is for annual checkups before you find yourself in pain.

"One joint dysfunctional and the whole musculoskeletal system will compensate," says the ACA's Jerome F. McAndrews, who notes that the pounding of physical-fitness-driven activity can exacerbate problems you don't even know you have. "Medical doctors and osteopaths will look at where you hurt and treat it. The chiropractor will wonder if the pain site is the original problem or if it's a sign of a compensation from a problem elsewhere."

Chiropractic manipulation or adjustment is the most common treatment, where a doctor uses his or her hands to apply pressure or physical thrust to a joint. And no, you don't necessarily have to hear a "snap," "crack," or "pop" in order for the treatment to be effective. Gentle movements can sometimes do the job just as well.

Although many medical insurance plans have yet to cover treatment from a D.C., the growing number of chiropractic enthusiasts might object to this being called an "alternative" form of care. Some indications of just how prevalent it's become: More than 40 percent of auto and 25 percent of on-the-job injuries of all kinds are treated in the D.C.'s office; the Agency for Health Care Policy and Research recommends chiropractic spinal manipulation as the safest, drug-free initial form of treatment for acute low-back problems in adults; and chiropractors serve on more than 150 hospital staffs.

McAndrews, like many others, is optimistic: "We're being called mainstream now."

Acupuncture/Acupressure

When President Richard Nixon visited China in 1972 and Beijing physicians eased his postsurgery abdominal pain with an exotic "needle therapy" called acupuncture, Americans seemed to suddenly discover one of the most ancient forms of healing there is.

Among the most thoroughly researched and documented alternative medical practices ever, acupuncture recently received the nod of a consensus panel convened by the NIH, which con-

SMART SOURCES

Acupuncture

National Alliance of Acupuncture and Oriental Medicine 14637 Starr Road South East Olalla, WA 98359 253-851-6895

F.Y.I.

Conventionally trained U.S. physicians who have taken courses to incorporate acupuncture in their medical practices 3,000*

Acupuncture practitioners in the United States 6,500*

Number of patient visits per year for acupuncture treatments . . . . . . 9–12 million**

Money spent on acupuncture in the United States, annually . . . . . . $500 million**

* Office of Alternative Medicine, National Institutes of Health

** U.S. Food and Drug Administration

cluded, "There is clear evidence that needle acupuncture treatment is effective" for a number of ills. Panel members even spoke up for increased insurance coverage to allow more people "public access" to its benefits.

The principle? Acupuncture and acupressure are, like reflexology and massage therapies, based on getting life energy—in this case called *qi* (pronounced "chee")—flowing right. Acupuncturists do this by gently inserting extremely fine needles in energy points that relate to vital organs and systems; acupressurists (like shiatsu practitioners) use pressure or massage; other, related practices employ heat, friction, suction, or impulses of electromagnetic energy.

Among other disorders, the techniques have been used to treat arthritis, headache, and depression, and reduce dependencies on everything from drugs and alcohol to cigarettes and food. Athletes are no strangers to this healing art.

Structural Integration/Rolfing

"When you come out of a Rolf session, you often come out very invigorated," says Karna Handy, of the Rolf Institute of Structural Integration. "Your body functions better, it works better, it's better aligned."

"Rolfing," a trademark for a system of soft-tissue manipulation and movement education, started out as the nickname for Rolfing Structural Integration, named after its developer, Ida P. Rolf, Ph.D.

"This is the gospel of Structural Integration," she wrote. "When the body gets working appropriately, the force of gravity can flow through. Then, spontaneously, the body heals itself."

Rolf, whose doctorate was in biochemistry, saw gravity as the strongest physical force with which the body has to deal, particularly the body's connective tissues, which physically support it and all its pieces and parts. While a healthy connective tissue (or myofascial) system is flexible, elastic, and resilient, Rolf followers say, the effects of gravity, injury, or unbalanced movement cause the body to shift to accommodate them, and that can ultimately lead to muscles that are chronically tense.

Rolf found that by manipulating the myofascial system, she could "organize the imbalances" and bring on healthy posture and structural change. The result: greater flexibility, a feeling of lightness and fluidity, better balance, increased breathing capacity, increased energy, and greater self-confidence—all that a right relation with gravity should be.

The Basic Ten series, also known as "the Recipe," involves ten hour-long sessions, during which the client lies on a table while the practitioner applies pressure with hands, arms, and sometimes elbows, keeping the relationship between tissue, respiration, nervous system responses, and organization in gravity in mind. The client's role: to "breathe into" the area being worked on, make small movements, and discuss with the trainer the patterns of movement and use of gravity involved.

"We've seen it help a wide variety of people," says Susan Melchior, director of the Guild for Structural Integration, which trains GSI practitioners in Ida Rolf's technique.

Look for the more than 950 certified Rolfers, plus GSI practitioners, similarly skilled Hellerworkers, and others for structural integration work.

SMART SOURCES

Structural Integration

The Guild for Structural Integration
P.O. Box 1559
Boulder, CO 80306
800-447-0150
303-447-0122
www.rolfguild.org

The Rolf Institute of Structural Integration
205 Canyon Blvd.
Boulder, Colo. 80302
800-530-8875
303-449-5903
www.rolf.org

SMART SOURCES

**Alexander
Technique**

North American Society
of Teachers of the
Alexander Technique
3010 Hennepin Ave. S.
Suite 10
Minneapolis, MN 55408
800-473-0620
www.prairienet.org/alex-
andertech/nastat1.html

Movement Therapies

Like touch therapies, movement therapies are based on the idea that our bodies start out healthy, and then we throw the proverbial monkey wrench into the works. While touch therapies right this wrong by palpating, pushing, rubbing, pressing, or otherwise maneuvering our tissue, muscle, or bones, the movement therapies teach us how to move and use our bodies in ways that can correct the harm.

With some approaches, you to do the movement; with others, a practitioner moves you to teach you how; others use a combination of the two.

Alexander Technique

Frederick Matthias Alexander started out as a Shakespearean orator but left his mark in the technique he developed after he got a case of chronic laryngitis and traced the cause to muscular tension.

Neither a treatment nor an exercise, the Alexander Technique has been called a re-education of body and mind. Based on a concept called "primary control," which focuses on the relationship between head and neck, it encourages a return to the body's natural poise and coordination, where processes work efficiently as an integrated, dynamic whole. The "student" plays an active role in learning how to do this, by gradually acquiring the skills it takes to correct the lifetime of nasty habits that cause physical and emotional stress.

Most often taught on an individual basis during thirty- to sixty-minute lessons, the technique cannot be conveyed without hands-on work, says practitioner Ron Dennis, Ed.D. "It's a one-on-one relationship between a teacher who is attempting to convey a skill and a student who's attempting to learn it."

The teacher will observe your posture and movement patterns and then, by placing his or her hands on your neck, shoulders, and back, pick up more information about your patterns of breathing and moving, and what you may need to do differently. A minimum of ten sessions are necessary, though twenty to thirty are recommended.

After one class, says Dennis, "a very typical reaction is the experience of lightness in movement; of lightness in themselves."

Feldenkrais Method

"Exercise alone isn't enough," writes Lawrence W. Goldfarb, Ph.D., of Mind in Motion, in Santa Cruz, California. "Most of us are unaware of how we move. We pay attention to where we are going or what we are doing, not to how we move."

The Feldenkrais (rhymes with "ice") Method teaches us how to do just that by becoming aware of how the body works. "It helps awareness so that you can perform at a higher level," says Debbie Ashton, M.S., a Knoxville-based practitioner who worked with the Olympic kayakers in the 1996 Games and has helped horseback riders and ski instructors, as well as exercise "civilians" of every stripe.

Its developer, Moshe Feldenkrais, D.Sc., was a Russian-born physicist, judo expert, mechanical engineer, and educator. He was familiar with psychology and neurophysiology, and he was the patentee of a number of sonar devices on the side. After crippling knee injuries, Feldenkrais taught himself to walk again.

SMART SOURCES

Feldenkrais Method

The Feldenkrais Guild of North America
524 Ellsworth St., S.W.
P.O. Box 489
Albany, OR 97321
800-775-2118
541-926-0981
www.feldenkrais.com

WHAT MATTERS, WHAT DOESN'T

What Matters

• A properly trained and certified practitioner.

• Treatment appropriate to your needs.

What Doesn't

• Using one method to the exclusion of others.

• Always doing things the old way.

The Feldenkrais Method was born, and with it a way to improve posture, balance, and breathing; enhance coordination and flexibility; and gain new patterns of thinking, to name a few. "The thing that's different is you learn to do things for yourself that are specific to you," says Ashton. "If you can prevent bad habits from accumulating, there's less wear and tear on your whole system."

Taught in group "Awareness Through Movement" classes, during which a teacher verbally leads a sequence of moves, or through individual "Functional Integration" lessons, in which the teacher guides your movements with his or her hands, Feldenkrais relies on gentle movement and directed attention to get its message across.

"Feldenkrais is gentle," writes Lawrence Goldfarb. "The idea is that you will change most easily if the new movements are more comfortable than the old ones. I like to say that our motto is 'No pain, more gain.'"

Weighing the Alternatives

Approaches that are off the beaten path can provide new and possibly better answers, from better warm-up and workout to better health all around. On the other hand, we tend to know a lot less about them and what they can do to—as well as for—us. Keep in mind the following:

• **Make sure it's appropriate for you.** Some approaches are better for some things than others—yoga, for instance, may be great for flexibility,

Health-Store Hype or Hope?

Botanical medicine, homeopathic remedies, herbs, and hormones: Whether they're being swallowed by the teaspoon, brewed by the tea cup, or absorbed through body oils, self-prescribed treatments popular at health-food stores today can do as much harm as abuse of any prescription drug.

Dietary supplements—including vitamins, minerals, and herbs—must meet the same Food and Drug Administration requirements as any food sold in the United States, but that doesn't mean that they're without risk. Certain portions of some herbs pose health dangers; others are dangerous when taken in megadose.

An Associated Press analysis of FDA records shows the agency has logged more than 2,500 reports of side effects and 79 deaths associated with supplements. About 900 of the illnesses and 44 deaths involved herbal products that contain ephedrine-like stimulants.

"Consumers seem to believe that any product that appears in pill form has been reviewed for safety by the FDA, which is not true for supplements," warns the Dietary Supplement Health and Education Act of 1994. And anyone with a history of disease or who is pregnant or nursing should not undertake *any* health-care agenda without professional care.

but a bad idea if you have any cardiac concerns. Decide what you want to get out of the experience, and find out if your expectations are in line.

• **Get references.** Talk with people who have been massaged, meditated, sat in "lotus position," or whatever you plan to do—preferably by the practitioner you plan to be doing it with. Scientific trials can provide solid clinical evidence of an approach's effects, but a personal view provides information you can't get from cold, hard stats.

• **Examine the practitioner.** If it's not conventional treatment, conventional rules and regulations are not going to be in place. Be sure the practitioner is licensed or regulated according to the laws of your state. Ask how long he's been in practice, what schools she's attended, what professional organizations he's a member of, what certifications she holds, and so on. A conventional variety of wide-ranging questions are your best bet.

• **Contact a national organization.** National groups familiar with state licensing, certification, and registration laws can often provide referrals and information about specific practitioners. Local and state health regulatory agencies and consumer affairs departments can also be helpful, and will inform you of any other clients' complaints.

• **Check out the office.** It won't tell you how effective or safe the treatment is, but it can matter when you're choosing who's practicing on you. Visit. Ask how many patients are typically seen in a day or week, and how much time the practitioner spends with each.

• **Consider the cost.** Many alternative treatments are not reimbursable by health insurance. Some are. Regulatory agencies and professional associations are good resources of what you might expect.

• **Ask your doctor or trainer.** Competent healthcare management requires knowledge of both conventional and alternative therapies for the practitioner to have a complete picture of your treatment plan.

THE BOTTOM LINE

For many, alternative approaches can provide the healing element of working out—not just by providing physical benefits and relief during times of injury, but by helping our minds and, dare we say, our spirits to be replenished as well. New applications of old tried-and-true methods, administered or led by trained professionals who know how, can add another dimension to healthy life.

....

Living the Fit Life

Our lives, lived well, are not confined to the four walls of a fitness center, or bound by an eat-at-home diet of fat-free cottage cheese. Fitness, done right, isn't either. Fitness fits in at the office, in the playground, at your favorite restaurant. All you need is the will to find the ways.

Working Out at Work

The salt mines. The grindstone. The office. The place where many of us spend a third of our lives, and where many of us can better our lives as well.

More than 81 percent of America's businesses with fifty or more employees have some kind of health-promotion program, according to the Wellness Councils of America (WELCOA), a national nonprofit group with a focus on healthier workplace lifestyles. The most popular: exercise, smoking cessation, back care, and stress management.

Altruism aside, keeping employees healthy is good for business, and the corporate world is encouraging the pursuit of fitness with workout breaks, team sports, and financial incentives, to name a few. Union Pacific Railroad's wellness program has gone so far as to convert old railroad cars into rolling fitness centers for distant workers' use.

"It's not really necessary for companies to have their own gym," says Angie Deming, WELCOA health educator. "Just offering a discount to a facility nearby is a great way to give employees the opportunity to improve fitness."

Meanwhile, as we spend more hours at work, on-the-job fitness routines make more and more sense. For one thing, we have less time to work out anywhere else. And, if the extent of your workday physical activity is limited to hefting a telephone receiver or swiveling a turn or two in that big leather chair, your body—and your mind—will crave a physical-activity break.

A wide range of strength and flexibility exercises can be done at your desk, while you're on the phone, even during that endless staff meeting. "Writing the alphabet" (rotating your foot to "write" each letter), heel lifts (pressing down on the toes for a few seconds while lifting the heel), or buttocks squeezes (momentarily tightening your "glutes"), can be done without anyone even knowing you're working out.

Other exercises—like desk push-ups, chest presses, and wall squats—are less inconspicuous but are still easy to do on-site. (If you don't have a set of handweights in your desk drawer, a book or paperweight can fill in as resistance in a crunch.) Stretches—including neck and shoulder rolls, shrugs and circles—reduce neck, shoulder, and back tension that come from sitting in place all day long. Repetitive hand movements such as those involved in a day of typing can cause painful carpal tunnel syndrome in hands and wrists: Flexes and extensions help, as will inexpensive "squeezies"—those sand- or grain-filled sacks so convenient for exercising the hand.

While you're at the keyboard, "don't stare at the computer screen too long," says Deming. Eyestrain, burning, dryness, watering, and blurred vision can result. Looking away every quarter hour or so, and slowly rolling the eyes in one direction, then the other, give them a workout.

And don't forget to get your aerobic activity in. Take the stairs instead of the elevator, use your

WHAT MATTERS, WHAT DOESN'T

What Matters

• Fitness that fits into your life.

• Tasty food in sensible portions, with healthy, smart preparation.

• Enjoyable and safe sporting, with helmets and protective gear.

What Doesn't

• A fitness regime that won't make it on the road.

• Self-deprivation in the name of health.

• Winning the game.

lunchtime for a change of scenery, walk to out-of-the-office meetings, and get away from the work site whenever you can.

Travel: How to Keep a Fitness Routine Going While You're Gone

Whether a trip is for business or pleasure, the demands of travel can be a workout in and of themselves. Run to catch your flight (aerobic), heft a suitcase (resistance), and wedge yourself into the standard airplane seat (flexibility, a.k.a. contortion), and you might feel as if you've covered all your bases, and more.

But if you're thinking that even the attempt to fit in some exercise basics will make an already tense on-the-go situation even worse, think again. Even a travel-sized portion of your fitness routine can reduce stress and is available most anywhere you go.

"There are more and more hotels that have fitness facilities," says Cathy Masterson McNeil, of the International Health, Racquet and Sportsclub Association. "Not just a fitness center, but a staffed fitness center."

Those that don't have facilities on-site will often have agreements with local clubs to allow guests free access (ask before making your reservation whether the gym the brochure includes among the amenities is on the premises or across town).

Some hotels even provide "fitness room service," delivering exercise videos and equipment from dumbbells to treadmills to your door; others will arrange for a personal trainer or, at the least, put you in touch with a nearby gym for a nominal visitors' fee. Alternatively, if you belong to a gym, ask if they have exchange or visitors' privileges anywhere near where you're going. And ask your trainer for a travel routine.

Staying with Aunt Lizzie, whose closest thing to gym equipment is a broken-down piece of lawn-care machinery in the garage? Walk her dogs, mow her lawn, help clean out that attic. . . . Not only will you accrue exercise benefits, but good-relative points as well. Pack a few of your own videos (if you have to, you can rent the VCR), a jump rope, and some portable free weights, like collapsible hand weights you can fill with water, or lightweight rubber resistance products like exercise bands, and you've got the makings of a health club to go.

And remember, wherever you're staying, you don't need a room full of equipment for a good workout. Tour the area or jog in place for your aerobics; practice your stretches to maintain flexibility; and hoist that nephew of yours for a few sets of resistance work. Bring a good pair of athletic shoes, comfortable clothing, and a Walkman, and you're set.

Three Good Gadgets

1. **"Squeezies."** Inexpensive sand- or grain-filled balls are great for exercising the hand.

2. **Telephone headsets.** Eliminate the need to hold the phone between ear and shoulder in a position favored only by muscle-tension enthusiasts.

3. **Padded wrist-rests.** Comfortably keep hands in proper position at the computer keyboard.

On Vacation

Healthy vacation options used to mean fat farms or taking the waters at a hard-to-find locale. Today, fitness camps and luxury health resorts cater to every whim, whether those whims involve becoming a marathon runner, or a massage-induced blob. With even travel expert Arthur

Sitting Down on the Job

As Mother always said, "Sit up straight and don't slouch. And keep those feet flat on the floor." Back pain is one of the most common medical problems around, and sitting improperly and for too long at a time are among its most common causes.

• **Get some support.** If your desk chair isn't one of those wonderful ergonomic models, keep your lower back supported with a small pillow, rolled towel, or seat support.

• **Chin up.** Keep your ears in line with your shoulders, and your chin parallel to the floor.

• **Pull in.** Sit close to the desk, with shoulders relaxed, upper arms vertical, forearms horizontal, and wrists in neutral position—neither turned in nor out, flexed nor extended. And if your chair has a swivel, use it—not your spinal column—for turns.

• **Make it easy on yourself.** Keep frequently used items—keyboard or phone—within reach. And when you lean forward at your desk, do so from the hips, not by rounding your back. If you insist on holding the phone between ear and shoulder—and you shouldn't—at least change off left and right.

• **Get up.** Every half hour or so, get up, take a walk, and give your back a break. And if you find yourself standing for long periods of time, keep your abs pulled in, your hips slightly tucked under, and your knees relaxed.

Frommer touting stays at yoga-centered ashrams, what were once considered esoteric vacation "alternatives" have become vacation mainstream.

High in the Canadian Rockies, the lavish surroundings of Solace, at the Banff Springs Hotel, frame cascading waterfall and mineral pools, while a state-of-the-art fitness center offers breathtaking mountain views. In the United States, enjoy a glimpse of what a $14,000 initiation fee can get you at the Houstonian Hotel, Club & Spa, in Texas, rated one of the nation's top ten health clubs and fitness centers by *Fitness* magazine. Access to the 125,000-square-foot members-only private club—with its 100-plus cardiovascular machines, rock-climbing wall, computerized indoor track, and Texas-big range of classes—is extended on a complimentary basis to all guests during their stay.

Spa-Finders and Resort2Fitness ("vacations for the mind, body, and spirit") are some of the specialists in the field. Whether you're looking for simple pampering, sports, the austerity of a no-frills Buddhist ashram, or ultra-deluxe accommodations to the tune of $4,000 or more per week (the grand suite at Grand Wailea on Maui costs $10,000 a night), there is a spa for you.

If you prefer your activity built into your vacation, rather than having it be the sole focus, just about any place plus a tour guide will do. Just stay off the tour bus, and see the sights by foot (or pedal, or flipper—as long as you provide the propulsion yourself). You'll get more of a workout, and you'll get more out of your tour. Sometimes the layout of your hotel will provide a jump start: With literally hundreds of steps from beachside to guest suites, gorgeous Anse Chastanet in St. Lucia, built into the side of a mountain, is the StairMaster of luxury resorts.

"Activity" or "adventure" vacations go a step—okay, a leap—beyond. Try mountain biking in Mongolia, skydiving in Las Vegas, bungy-jumping in New Zealand, or trekking the Himalayas in Nepal. Beginners might feel more comfortable with, say, cycling over the flatlands, or any one of numerous other less strenuous but still physically active tours. Even the "gentle" walking promised

Eating En Route

Although we've a way to go before we'll extol the virtues of airline food, there are ways to reserve a healthier, perhaps more palatable repast. Many airlines offer special meals that you can order ahead. Delta's choices include Kosher, Asian, Hindu, and Muslim meals; those that are gluten-free, low-fat, low-sodium, or low-calorie; a fruit plate, and two types of vegetarian.

As in any restaurant situation, the farther you are from hunger, the easier it will be to resist temptations on a tray-table so close to your mouth. Have a piece of fruit or a cup of low-fat yogurt before you're buckled into your seat belt, and unload any danger foods into the airsickness bag.

As far as what's available in the airport itself, the American Dietetic Association is optimistic about the growing variety of healthy food options. An ADA survey of twenty-eight major airports nationwide found improvements over a similar survey a few years before. All offered fresh fruit and fruit juices, and nearly all had bagels, pretzels, salads, and low-fat or nonfat yogurt; eleven had salad bars.

"We were pleased that with a little effort, we could find a wide selection of healthful food choices in most airports," said ADA spokesperson Cathy Kapica, Ph.D., R.D.

A few have special play areas for kids to burn energy while waiting, and whatever your age, a walk before or after your flight is a good idea—not only to scout out your food options, but for the exercise benefits as well. Walk from Terminal 1 to Terminal 3 at Chicago's O'Hare International Airport, and you'll cover about 1.25 miles, and 150 calories.

In the airplane or in the terminal, remember the fail-safe alternative: Bring your own.

by Wings, an international birdwatching tour group based in Tucson, can last up to six hours, and be modified for faster and slower groups.

GreenTracks, in Durango, Colorado, offers nature-oriented forays into tropical regions, while a little-known University of Nevada web site (www.nscee.edu/unlv/Colleges/College_of_Hotel_Admin/Tourism/adv.html) lists an amazing array of links. The twice-annual Specialty Travel Index (also available at www.spectrav.com) lists tour operators for more than 150 special interests, from aerobics to zoology. Then there's the second childhood option: "Go to camp. Be a kid again," says coach Roy T. Benson, president of Running, Ltd. camps. "Baseball, soccer, there's a camp for everything."

A word of caution: Before you put down a deposit anywhere, find out what condition you're expected to be in, and believe it. And for business or pleasure, of whatever kind, if you travel to a higher altitude, take it easy. With thinner air up there, you'll be breathing harder even at rest.

Restaurant Smarts: Strategies to Stay on Track

Eating out, taking out, or ordering in—we Americans are purchasing more of our meals than we ever have before. About 40 percent of all food dollars are spent on food prepared away from our own kitchens, accounting for a significant proportion of the calories we eat. And a significant impact on our health.

What Sports, Where

The National Sporting Goods Association took a look at sports participation in major metropolitan areas. Here, the most popular in ten of them:

Atlanta: Tennis

Boston: Salt-water fishing

Chicago: Volleyball

Detroit: Bowling

Houston: Salt-water fishing

Los Angeles/Long Beach: Horseback riding

New York: Calisthenics

Philadelphia: Downhill skiing

Riverside/San Bernadino: Table tennis

Washington, D.C./Baltimore: Tennis

Just as the Food and Drug Administration regulates claims on food labels, it now regulates the terms restaurants use to describe their meals. "The idea is for the claims to mean the same thing wherever they show up—on food labels in the store or on menus in a restaurant," said a food technologist in the FDA's Office of Food Labeling.

Restaurants can promote their fare using nutrient claims (for example, "low fat" or "high fiber") or health claims, which refer to the link between a nutrient or food and a disease or health condition. A dish that's low in fat, saturated fat, and cholesterol, and provides significant amounts of one or more of the key nutrients vitamins A and C, iron, calcium, protein, and fiber, might be able to carry a claim about how diets low in saturated fat and cholesterol may reduce the risk of heart disease. In those cases, look for "heart healthy," "heart smart," or simply a picture of a heart.

"Light" means the item has fewer calories and less fat than the food to which it's being compared, unless portion size is the factor, in which case the restaurant has to say so. "Healthy" means the item is low in fat and saturated fat, has limited amounts of cholesterol and sodium, and provides significant amounts of one or more of the six key nutrients.

If you want specific information related to the

claims, the restaurant is obliged to provide it, but they're not obliged to stand up to laboratory analyses for accuracy. "It should be accurate," said that same food technologist, "but not necessarily precise."

To that, we say get your handy pocket calorie-counter food guide and pack it with you before you go. Here are a few other tips:

• Avoid high-fat toppings that can "undo" even low-fat foods: On baked potatoes, skip the cheese, bacon, and sour cream toppings in favor of salsa, low-fat dressing, or yogurt.

• Don't be tempted by the menu. Keep it closed, and order what you want.

• Try one or two appetizers and a side salad instead of an entree.

• Avoid all-you-can-eats.

• Alcohol is high in calories and lowers your resistance. If you must, drink it with (not before) your meal to cut absorption, and order by the glass.

• Trim all visible fat from meat, and remove breading and skin.

• Speak up. Ask for meals to be prepared to your specifications, such as with olive or canola oil instead of butter or margarine.

Exercise Is for All!

America's favorite sport activities and their participants (in millions):

Individual sports

Bowling 52.2

Billiards 44.5

In-line skating 27.5

Water sports

Swimming (fitness) 23.0

Water skiing 9.6

Scuba diving 2.4

Winter sports

Downhill skiing 13.7

Cross-country skiing 4.0

Snowboarding 3.2

Team sports

Basketball 45.6

Volleyball
(hard surface) 26.4

Softball (fast
and slow pitch) 25.3

Source: Sporting Goods Manufacturers Association

SMART MONEY

"Don't hide good food," says Kristine Clark, director of sports nutrition at the Center for Sports Medicine at Penn State University. "People buy fruits and vegetables with good intentions and put them in drawers in their refrigerators and forget they're there." Keep the good stuff visible, in countertop baskets or on eye-level refrigerator shelves. Stash the beer, soda, and dessert items out of sight.

• Watch for large serving sizes. Split your portion with your dining companion, or ask your server to pack half the meal before you start.

• Have bread and butter or chips removed from the table or served during your meal.

• Be suspicious of salads. Chef's salad contains cheese, eggs, and high-fat meats.

• Request sauces and salad dressings on the side, then dip your fork into the sauce or dressing first, before spearing your food.

Know Substitutions

• Skim or low-fat milk instead of whole milk, cream, or half-and-half.

• Chicken, turkey, or seafood instead of red meat.

• Salad, vegetables, rice, pasta, or baked potato instead of French fries.

• Fresh fruit or sorbet instead of sugary high-fat desserts.

• Jam or margarine instead of butter.

• Egg substitutes or egg whites instead of whole eggs.

• Whole-grain breads and rolls or breadsticks instead of muffins or croissants.

• Mustard, salsa, or barbecue sauce instead of mayonnaise or "special" sandwich sauce.

• Leaner cuts such as sirloin, tenderloin, and flank steak instead of fatty prime cuts of meat.

• Grilled onions and mushrooms instead of bacon, cheese, or sour cream.

Eat the Pickles, Eat the Lettuce . . .

But hold all that special sauce.

Fast food is as much of an American classic as our high blood pressure. Next on the list, our penchant for eating out on Chinese. And Italian. And Mexican. Here's a rundown on what to eat at our favorite eateries.

Chinese

Does Chinese deserve its time-honored reputation for being more healthful than what we hamburger-flipping Americans usually eat?

Yes. And no.

Like Indian, Thai, Japanese, and other Asian cuisine, the Chinese menu offers many lower-fat poultry, seafood, vegetable, and noodle dishes; goes relatively light on the pork and beef; and favors stir-frying over deep-frying of foods. And we challenge you to find anything involving cheese. The result is saturated fat generally lower than you'd find in the typical American meal.

Of course, batter-dipped sweet-and-sour pork, things called "crispy," and Japanese tempuras are just some of the exceptions to prove the rule. Then there are those egg rolls in fried wrappers; nut-riddled, sauce-heavy "special" dishes; and

"Eating out and eating 'ethnic' foods while you're away from home doesn't have to be detrimental to your nutritional plan," says Tony Clark, a thirty-three-year-old publishing professional in New York City. "I try to enjoy the foods of the places I'm visiting. I usually get in a good deal of physical activity when on vacation—in sightseeing and walking. And enjoying something that I wouldn't normally have at home is a pleasure. You should never feel you've deprived yourself, especially when on vacation. Set some parameters for comfortable, allowable weight *gain* during vacations—say two or three pounds. Then when you return, go right back to your fitness and nutrition program. The key is to enjoy yourself at *all* times."

meals with higher sodium content than a salt shaker might hold. And stir-frying, while better than deep-frying, is still frying. Steamed or braised is a more healthful choice.

Eating your Chinese food Chinese-style can help. Order a big bowl of steamed rice, and instead of having the rice sop up the sauce on your plate, work the other way around by bringing your food out of the sauce and to the rice. If you're hooked on fried rice, ask that the chef leave out the egg, and mix your order with steamed rice to lessen the damage. Other special requests can include low-sodium soy sauce on the table, a limit on the nuts included in your dish, and a larger portion of vegetables than meat. An order of steamed vegetables is a good accompaniment to any meal; the more you fill up on rice and steamed veggies, the less sodium and fat you'll be taking in. And you still won't be hungry a half hour after you eat.

Italian

The good news about Italian food is the good effect a Mediterranean diet can have on health: lower rates of heart disease, colon cancer, and obesity, to name a few. The important news is that this doesn't happen automatically when you walk inside the local trattoria. The choices you make while you're in there do play a part.

Go for the pasta and bread, vegetables and legumes, olive oil and fruits like those long-lived southern Italians do, with their minimal use of meat, and you'll be on the right track. (Veal parmigiana and cannolis, on the other hand, will derail you every time.)

Eating family-style is a good idea. If your

entree isn't accompanied by a side dish of pasta, order at least one to be shared; like the rice in Chinese restaurants, it's great to help cut fat and keep you full. A moderate-size slice of Italian bread also helps—but not if it's a slab of garlic bread slathered with butter and cheese. If you must, dip plain bread in a little olive oil, and sprinkle with a pinch of Parmesan.

Aside from choosing vegetables, seafood, or chicken over the red meat and veal, you can improve the health value of your selection with the choice of sauce. The best: meatless, tomato-based marinara, lowest in fat of all. The worst: butter, cream, or cheese sauces like Alfredo, and those containing greater amounts of meat. Pesto and tomato sauces offer a happy medium.

On pizza, as with other fare, the danger lurks in the cheeses and meats—especially fatty sausage, bacon, and pepperoni. Ask for less cheese and more vegetables. Or skip the cheese altogether and order a pesto pie.

Mexican

If only the rice and beans served south of the border were as good for us as they sound. But, like other side dishes popular at America's favorite cantinas, they're filled with fat and sodium to spare. Combine them with the sour cream, guacamole, and the basket of tortilla chips, and you can get your fill without even touching that cheese-filled, batter-dipped, deep-fried chile relleno you crave.

But don't despair; there are options. Beans that aren't refried are a beginning, or better yet, order à la carte and avoid both them and the rice. Push the tortilla chips, sour cream, and guacamole to the end of the table (or ask the waiter to remove them), and keep the flavorful yet fat-free salsa or pico de gallo nearby.

Everyone's favorites—enchiladas, chimichangas, and tacos—present another challenge if you're trying to eat for health. Made mostly of corn- or white-flour tortillas, they can be stuffed with any of a variety of ingredients, and what you choose to have them stuffed with—beef, vegetables, and any combination of the omnipresent rice, beans, and cheese—counts. Preparation does, too. Some are cooked in oil (enchiladas), deep-fried (hard tacos), or immersed in boiling oil, filling and all (chimichangas). Fajitas, burritos, quesadillas, and soft tacos are spared.

Your best bet: the seafood, chicken, or vegetable fajitas, as long as you don't go *loco* on toppings of the cardio-loading kind.

Fast Food

Even at fast-food restaurants, there's hope. Although many "lite" menus have given way to heavier selections, grilled chicken, pitas, and salads offer McChoice. The key to healthier eating is, as always, to have it your way:

Rule 1: In general, avoid anything involving the word "deluxe."

Rule 2: Stay away from things hidden beneath "crispy golden" coatings.

Rule 3: Choose toppings with care.

A stuffed pita pocket or flour tortilla containing salad, chicken, or fish can usually beat a burger healthwise, but make sure you know what's in there: Vegetables and rice are great; heavy cheese or sauce will undo your good intentions.

Grilled or baked chicken sandwiches have become popular menu choices. Grilled and baked are good. Chicken is good. But grilled or baked chicken with fattening sauces or mayo aren't. Opt for light dressing, mustard, or barbecue sauce. Light subs, especially on whole-grain breads if you can find them, are best topped with onions (not sautéed), tomatoes, and peppers, with a whole lot of lettuce for crunch.

Main- or side-order salads teamed with a baked potato can add up to a satisfying meal, even if there's not much in that salad vegetable-wise. Get your broccoli on the potato, hold off on the cheese-color topping it's usually drenched with, and use a low-fat dressing on both.

Many calorie-counting, nutrition-tallying books can give you name-brand information. For cyber types, Olen Publishing's interactive "Food Finder" will tell you about more than a thousand fast-food items, from Arby's to White Castle, at www.olen.com/food. Based on the handbook *Fast Food Facts* by the Minnesota Attorney General's Office, it allows you to type in the restaurant, food, and maximum number of calories, fat, cholesterol,

Menuspeak

As a quick way to gauge the fat content of your restaurant meal, watch for these words:

Low-Fat Words	High-Fat Words
au jus	Alfredo
au vin	au gratin
baked	basted
balsamic	batter-dipped
braised	béarnaise
broiled	béchamel
consommé	beurre blanc
dry rub	bordelaise
en brochette	breaded
fresh	buttery
fruit glaze	creamed
fruit-sweetened	crème fraîche
grilled	crispy
herb-crusted	croissant
light	en casserole
marinara	en croûte
marinated	filo wrapped
oil-free	fried
poached	gravy
red sauce	hollandaise
roasted	parmigiana
steamed	puff pastry
stir-fried in broth	rich
tomato-based	sautéed
vegetable-based	scalloped
vinaigrette	stir-fried in oil
whole-grain	stuffed
yogurt	tempura

or sodium you want in it. Print it out and you have a glove-compartment-convenient guide.

Never Too Young: Working Baby into Your Workout

According to the American Medical Association, even a newborn, just beginning to develop motor skills, can benefit from a baby-size workout, with Mom or Dad gently cycling his arms or legs as he lays on his back. The AMA recommends that once the baby is one to three months old, you play simple games like "Fly Baby Fly": Sit on the floor with baby facing you; support her body with your hands around her chest and under her arms; and, with a big "Wheee!" lift the baby as you gently roll onto your back and hold her up high.

Exercising with your children when they are young may well be the best way to ingrain the habit. In addition to the physical benefits they'll reap, there are definite psychological benefits as well. And it's not bad for Mom and Dad to join in the family fun, either.

To find a class, contact your gym, doctor, hospital, place of worship, or local YM/YWCA. New moms and pregnant women should be sure that the class meets the American College of Obstetricians and Gynecologists exercise guidelines, and that the (appropriately certified) instructor is properly trained to work with different fitness levels. Check with your (and your baby's) physician before starting any exercise plan.

THE BOTTOM LINE

On the job, at play, wherever we are and whoever we're with, fitness fits in. Not to be confined to a gym or a treadmill, or tolerated like a dose of distasteful medicine at a prescribed time or place, fitness—done right—is a thing to be enjoyed. It's the only way you're likely to want it, and it's the only way it will work. So find an activity you like; grab a friend, family member, or your dog to share in it; and live lively, live long . . . live fit!

Index

Books in the
Smart Guide™ Series

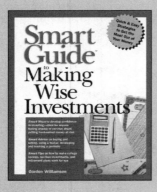

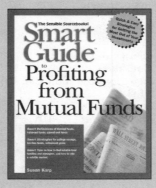

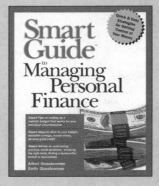

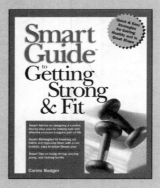

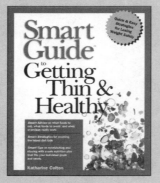

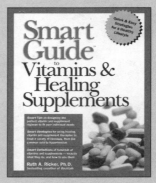

Smart Guide™ to
Getting Strong and Fit

Smart Guide™ to
Getting Thin and
Healthy

Smart Guide™ to
Making Wise
Investments

Smart Guide™ to
Managing Personal
Finance

Smart Guide™ to
Profiting from Mutual
Funds

Smart Guide™ to
Vitamins and Healing
Supplements

Available soon:

Smart Guide™ to
Boosting Your Energy

Smart Guide™ to
Healing Foods

Smart Guide™ to
Home Buying

Smart Guide™ to
Relieving Stress

Smart Guide™ to
Starting and Operating
a Small Business

Smart Guide™ to
Time Management